My Angel Andrei

My Angel Andrei

Antoinette Romero

Writer's Showcase
San Jose New York Lincoln Shanghai

My Angel Andrei

Writer's Showcase
an imprint of iUniverse.com, Inc.

For information address:
iUniverse.com, Inc.
5220 S 16th, Ste. 200
Lincoln, NE 68512
www.iuniverse.com

ISBN: 0-595-18831-1

Printed in the United States of America

*A memoir of a child's struggle with cancer and
a mother's struggle to survive the loss*

Dedication

This book is dedicated to my beautiful, loving child and loving family. Life's experiences teach us to appreciate and value life to the fullest because it is up to us to make a difference when these lessons touch our souls. My lessons learned would have never been possible without my family's love, faith, tenderness and positive attitude toward everything.

Contents

Acknowledgments

I would like to acknowledge the immense help given to me in completing this book. I wish to thank my mother and father, Antoinette and Francisco Romero; my sister, Linda Romero Shah; brother, Frank Romero; and nephew, Augustine Romero, for all of their loving support and the courage they all exemplified that allowed me to succeed in becoming a survivor.

I also wish to thank Navid Daniel Rastein, M.D. for all his help in accomplishing my dream; Rosemary Colgrove, for her caring friendship and assistance throughout this book; and to Kamran Harsini for being my confidante and the special friendship we share; and to all my dear friends who have blessed this book with their good wishes and encouragement not to give up on something that was so sacred and significant to me. Believing in me helped me believe in myself. Thank you professor Dr. Blaise Bonpane, you inspired me after reading an essay I wrote for your class, to write a book about my experience.

I would also like to thank the most precious person who made this experience, growth and spiritual awakening possible: my "Angel Andrei." Thank you for the great satisfaction and honor of being your mother.

May your wings keep flying above with a sweet smile knowing your mommy believes your life and death was not in vain.

Introduction

For me, life has been very difficult and I have suffered an enormous loss. I will never be the same person again, there is an immense emptiness in my heart. However, although I will never be whole again and my heart will never completely heal, I am proud to be the person I am now. I would go through it all again to have been as blessed and fortunate as I was to be Andrei's mommy.

My beautiful, handsome and courageous child was diagnosed with a malignant brain tumor at the age of two-and-a-half and lived to the age of three-and-a-half. He left behind many remarkable memories, in particular, he taught me to become a courageous woman, to become a survivor in a world in which he would no longer be physically with me.

We both loved, learned, taught and held on to each other during his short time on earth. The final year of his life was obviously the most essential. We went through chemotherapy, radiation, surgeries and we gave each other the strength to finally let go at the end of this journey but only to begin a new journey in our lives. Andrei is in Heaven with God, watching over his loved ones and he's no longer in pain or suffering. I honestly believe that beauty, love and an endless peace surround him.

My journey exists with God, family and friends, with strength, courage and the will to continue on with the unforgettable memories we shared, and that I may share with others our emotions so that his time on this earth was not in vain. I believe there's a reason for certain experiences we must encounter, although sad, something good must be learned from that experience. Parents whose children may be stricken with cancer can learn the significance of survival through my personal experience and the gift of life.

Chapter 1
Age of Innocence

When we're young and naïve about life, we have no clue about what the future and destiny hold for us. Of course, we would rather live life day to day, not knowing what is expected, especially if it's tragic and painful.

I became involved in a relationship with a gentleman from my job who, while we were dating, was a kind, goodhearted and sincere guy. His name is Sebastian Carrillo. I was a very innocent, naïve girl and a virgin.

I did not fall in love with Sebastian immediately but I worked with him side by side, late hours during the night. Somehow, one day, I fell head over heels in love with him, so much so that my strong religious beliefs and convictions were no longer a priority. His pale skin, black hair and hazel eyes dazzled me. I felt very deeply within my heart that this would be the man I would marry and raise children with. Sebastian felt the same, however, he was not completely ready to commit at the age of nineteen. He still needed to experience his youth and freedom.

The first year we were pretty content as boyfriend and girlfriend, we loved each other deeply. One thing that remains clear in my mind was when we discussed and fantasized about the baby we would have one day, we even named him Jr. for Sebastian junior. I would frequently receive love notes or postcards from Sebastian with P. S. remarks reading, "Say hi to Jr. for me." We would actually envision ourselves with our future baby boy that we would one day conceive and be wonderful parents to.

The day I turned twenty, Sebastian gave me a promise ring. When he put it on my finger, he confessed tearfully the enormous love he felt for me. Sebastian began discussing marriage even though we felt we were young to marry. He was going with his emotions. We decided to wait since he was attending college at the same time.

We spent every moment together. We both worked for a foreign national airline in the evenings at the Los Angeles International Flights Division. During the day we spent even more time together, enjoying precious moments. We attended live concerts, went to the beach and rode bicycles. We were very happy.

After a year, our relationship began to get rocky. At the time, the company was closing down its reservations department and centralizing it in Miami. People with more seniority would be able to bump the airport personnel; I became affected and was furloughed. I had the option to bump another person in the different states where we were based, but I declined.

The separation from working together put a damper on our relationship. Many of the guys who bumped and transferred to the airport were single. Sebastian began to spend a lot of time with them and less with me. He was going out with his new friends more often and putting me aside. The lying began then and so did the cheating. He still loved me but not like I deserved to be loved. I felt it was a phase he was going through, and it would all change when he got tired of that lifestyle and appreciated what he and I had. Sebastian kept returning, stating he loved me and could never compare me to anyone else, because to him I was so pure and unique.

It's funny when I think about it now, because he often would repeat to me, "If I could only put you away in a refrigerator and freeze you just like you are and then, when I am ready to settle down, take you out just like you are. Perfect and beautiful, but a couple of years from now."

I allowed myself to remain in this confusing relationship; I was so blindly in love that my dignity was non-existent. I just assumed it would go away and things would be as they used to be. I had no experience; Sebastian was my first serious relationship and I was in love.

We stopped seeing each other when I discovered he was going out with a girl from work. I became very depressed. Everything that was so wonderful about this relationship had changed. During this tumultuous time, I felt trapped and wanted to get away. I sat with my parents and Lourdes, a co-worker and friend who came over to visit with her husband, Roberto, to sway my parents into allowing me to transfer temporarily to New Orleans. They explained to my parents that they would take care of me.

My parents felt my enthusiasm to continue working. I also insisted that I would lose my seniority if I did not continue working and, if positions re-opened, I would not qualify before the others. I loved my job, it gave me many opportunities to fly and see other countries. It has been my dream to travel and the opportunity was there with all the benefits you earn when you work for an airline. I felt the experience would be good for me. I wanted to grow and was not that frightened about the change since I was going to be living with a family, Roberto and Lourdes and their two children, Jennifer and Jonathan. My mother later confessed to me that she knew that I just wanted to be away from Sebastian and deal with my emotions from far away. She was right, I also wanted to prove to him that I was fine and moving on with my life.

My parents gave me their blessing and I started packing for New Orleans. When my parents took me to the airport, they looked sad and Mother embraced me and began to weep. I held back the tears so that it would not be so emotional. When the aircraft began to push back, I began crying. It was a tremendous step forward. My parents sheltered me and I loved them for trying to protect me so much, however, I needed to grow and expand. I felt that I needed to get away so that I may gain my sanity back.

During my time away, my mother was diagnosed with an illness that could leave her blind. My family didn't tell me the whole truth for fear of upsetting me; they wanted to wait until I returned for a visit to explain. My mother prohibited my family and friends to say anything to me. My friend, Marina, and a couple of other friends came to visit me with the plan that I return to Los Angeles with them for a short visit. I had already been away for three months. Apparently, Marina knew what was going on with my mother, but she respected my mother's wishes to keep silent. My mother's love is so unconditional and unselfish that she had told Marina she wanted me to enjoy my friends' visit and not be sad with her news. I flew back with them and, oddly enough, my family was not at the airport. Instead, Marina insisted on driving me home.

When I got out of the car, she embraced me as though I needed a hug for what was ahead of me. I walked towards the door where my whole family awaited my arrival. My brothers and sister-in-laws hugged and kissed me. Then Dad came and hugged and kissed me, followed by my sister and grandmother. During all this I am wondering, "Where is my mom?"

It was like a slow motion scene. After everyone welcomed me back, out of the right-hand corner of my eye, I finally saw my mother, crying and extending both arms out to me, speaking to me in Spanish. I ran to her, kneeled at her feet and we both embraced and cried. That is when reality struck; my mother was blind!

After hours of talking, I was told that she had been taking a medication called Coumadin, a drug that thins the blood. Apparently she experienced a hemorrhage and she suffered a detached retina. The day I said good-bye to my mother at Los Angeles Airport was the last time she ever saw my face.

I requested a month's leave of absence to nurse my mother after surgery scheduled for the next week. After five hours of surgery, the doctor informed us that my mother would never see again. The damage was so severe to the retina that it could not be repaired. It all felt like a nightmare.

Sebastian knew that I was back in Los Angeles. During this difficult time, I was heartbroken and lonely and really needed him to assist me through the pain. He sent a card telling me he was truly sorry for the tragedy my family and I were going through. He insisted on staying away so as not to make things harder for me since we were no longer seeing each other.

At the end of the month, I had return to New Orleans. My family and I had accomplished a lot. Mother did not want to go out in public, she was embarrassed and felt inadequate. We insisted on taking her out frequently to dinner and shopping malls, and assisted her in becoming acquainted with her home environment. Mother is a very strong woman and she dealt with her situation bravely.

I flew back to New Orleans and commuted on weekends to Los Angeles to care for my mother. I just worked Monday through Friday, flying back to Los Angeles Friday evenings and returning Monday morning at 6:00 a.m. I did this for eight more months until finally I was transferred to Los Angeles permanently. I was thrilled to be back home again and to be able to care for my mother who needed and missed me.

Chapter 2

Conception and Turmoil

Returning to Los Angeles had me working side by side with Sebastian again. I had made up my mind I would not go back to him and would continue with the goals that I had begun to focus on during my time away. I was a bit more mature and grounded. But working with Sebastian again was a strange feeling, and my emotions were confused.

The cycle began again two months after I started working with him. My involvement was off and on. I tried dating other people just as friends, not even being kissed by anyone. When Sebastian would see me meeting anyone at work or trying to get to know me better, he would try to get back together with me. He didn't want to lose me, but would not let go either. My being "hopelessly in love," but not fully committed, how very convenient for him. Somehow, I got caught up with every-thing again and my love for him was still very strong. I lost many opportunities to have an honest, dedicated relationship. I never permit-ted myself the chance to find happiness in another relationship that would complete me. I continued seeing Sebastian as if I did not deserve better, restrained to his conditions.

Soon I became pregnant. Amazingly enough, he was excited and looking forward to the baby's birth. I, on the other hand, was frantic; what would my parents and family think? I have been raised Catholic, in mostly Catholic schools, in a traditional Hispanic family. I am the youngest of five children and my parents expected me to get married the traditional way in a Catholic Church and definitely *not* pregnant.

I sat with Sebastian one day to discuss our situation. For the first time I was not so afraid and felt it would be okay. He told me he loved me and would take care of the baby and me. He said we would get married and that no one would know that I was pregnant. He only wanted his parents to know the truth, not mine since it would break their hearts. They would know after the wedding. I bought a wedding magazine to choose my dress and began discussing the wedding plans with my parents. Mother was not too thrilled since she had seen me suffer in this relationship but ultimately wanted me to be happy. She knew I loved Sebastian very much.

Sebastian and I were going to go out to dinner because he was going to make it special and propose officially. That night he called and said he needed to postpone it because it was the day he wanted to explain to his parents what was happening. I understood and expected him to call me the next night to inform me what had happened. After that is when all hell broke loose!

Sebastian was confused, undecided and tried avoiding me. The only time I would see him was at work and he could not avoid me. At that point, I figured that his parents had confused him with his decision and advised him not to rush into marriage. His parents did not dislike me; they disliked the fact that their youngest son, who was never allowed to take any responsibility for his actions, had to do so now.

This was something to be handled between Sebastian and myself. We were two adults who had to take some sort of responsibility for our actions. An unborn baby coming into this world has to be loved and wanted by both parents, regardless of any faults and immaturity.

Among all the turmoil, my mother came into my room one day and found me crying. That must have been one of the most difficult times of my life. She consoled me and said, "Don't cry, if he does not want to marry you, it's better this way. You will meet someone someday."

I turned to her and said, "You don't understand, Mom, I am pregnant."

I remember her placing her hands on her face and crying, "No, this can't be."

I begged her not to tell my dad until I thought things through. My mother was so distraught and devastated and the word "abortion" came up. It would facilitate removing the problem and responsibility I would encounter as a single parent, also nobody would have to find out.

We immediately went to St. Peter & St. Paul Church to speak to a priest. Soon Father Sean Cronin walked in, the priest who would play such an enormous part in the lives of my family, unborn child and myself.

My mother and I wept and told the priest I was about two months pregnant and the father was having second thoughts about marrying me. Father Cronin told me in his British, almost angelic voice, how blessed I was and that God had gifted me in having a child. His words consoled us and reaffirmed our religious beliefs. My mother was going to stand by and support me; she embraced me and I felt her warmth and protection.

Although abortion was mentioned, I know I would never contemplate it nor would my mother permit it. I became aware that I would probably experience humiliation from people by having a child out of wedlock. There was going to be pressure, stress and an incredible responsibility to raise a child on my own. But, deep down inside, I felt and knew in my heart I was pregnant with a baby who was part of Sebastian and myself. The love I had was worth the challenges and accountability that were ahead of me.

When we arrived home, Sebastian's sister Yolanda, called to insist I come over to discuss what she had just found out. My mother went with me, and I am so glad she insisted on coming because, to my surprise, his mother Maria Carrillo and his sister-in-law, Loretta were all anxious to express their opinion. After an hour of arguing, nothing was resolved.

Days later, Sebastian did a disappearing act from work and I didn't see or talk to him until about two weeks later.

Father Sean Cronin asked to speak to Sebastian and he agreed. I decided to wait for him outside the church so that he could feel free to express his emotions. When Sebastian left he approached me, hugged and kissed me, and told me he realized he loved me very much.

Looking straight into my eyes, he said, "I could never leave you. I love you very much and would feel like a dog if I ever left you."

He told me to please allow him some time to get his mind in order and we would be just fine. He also told me to go home and tell my parents things would be fine. It would be just a matter of time.

Obviously I came home thrilled and with a sense of peace of mind, since the secret was not out yet. Mom kept the secret with me to give Sebastian time to make things right.

Oddly enough, every time he would go home and speak to his parents his attitude changed tremendously, and he was no longer convinced of what he thought he wanted or felt. I don't want to put all the blame on Sebastian's parents. I believe Sebastian's own convictions should have been enough. How could I have expected him to have those convictions when we learn most of what we know and do from our role models, our parents?

During the following weeks, I finally realized that I could no longer continue in this agony of waiting. I finally gave Sebastian an ultimatum. Maybe, I should have given him space and waited. But I was immature and really could not come to terms with being a single parent. I was confused, scared and aware of the enormous responsibility of bringing another human being into this life. I thought I would gain more by pressuring him, all it did was frighten him more and allowed him the easy way out, which is precisely what he acted upon.

Since we could no longer keep up the front, my mother and I decided to tell the family. Everyone was informed of my pregnancy. They hugged me, reassured me of the love and support they would share with my unborn baby and me. Their attitude and response gave me courage and strength to face what the future held for us; little did I know that it was going to be greater than I imagined.

I continued working, Sebastian by my side, some days wanting to be a part of my life, other times pulling away. His family decided never to speak to me again. His sister, who worked for the same company, would see me at certain functions or meetings and completely ignore my existence.

I had an extremely difficult pregnancy, constantly crying, watching Sebastian flirt with other women at work. He took trips; he purchased a sports car and always had a big smile at work gatherings and holiday celebrations. He ignored the actual truth of dealing with our situation and acted like it was not difficult.

My friend, Lourdes, was always the main person who kept communication flowing between Sebastian and myself. I would express to her how upset he was making me. She would talk to him and try to make him understand, at times it worked but it would only last for a short period of time and he would continue being careless and unemotional to my feelings.

My other dear friend, Cassandra, would also get involved frequently.

One day he told her he doubted if this was his child. She told him how could he have the audacity to even think that when he knew how much I loved him, and I had never been with another man. I also heard this kind of suggestion through his parents' friends.

I never imagined Sebastian would be so cowardly, he was someone so different from the man I had fallen in love with. He had changed and it was for the worst. I was told that his parents were telling their friends that he was not living up to his responsibility because it was not his child. His parents' friends did not believe them because they had befriended me throughout the years and obviously had a very authentic perception of how genuinely honest and pure my love was for Sebastian. This was just another way of protecting and sheltering their son from responsibility and keeping a nice image among their family and friends.

At times I would lock myself in my bedroom and cry. My brother, Gerald, would stand by the door and say, "Sis, don't cry, it's not good for the baby. Sebastian's not worth it, take care of yourself and, when the baby's born, everything will feel fine."

Gerald was a great emotional support. Towards the last months of my pregnancy, my eldest brother, Augustine, would bring me lunch everyday: shakes and dill pickles in particular. Emotionally I had my ups and downs, but my whole family was extremely supportive and caring. With the help of my family, I began to purchase the crib and set up the room to accommodate the baby and me. My due date was approaching, January 7, 1987.

My co-workers gave me a surprise baby shower at the office and many gifts were bestowed, such as the bassinet, car seat and clothes. My mother and sister, Linda, were also invited to the surprise party, I cried when I walked in. To my disbelief, Sebastian appeared briefly and this allowed him the opportunity to make amends with two of my family members. His sister, Yolanda, had a great relationship with me prior to my becoming pregnant since we both worked for the same company. However, now she ignored me at work and also did not attend the baby shower. Sebastian left the party abruptly without any explanation and left me to find a way to take home the many gifts.

Ironically, two years before, Yolanda became pregnant by a guy who resided in Mexico whom she had briefly met on a trip to Cancun. Yet Sebastian's parents did not want him to leave their daughter in that condition, that was not acceptable to them. He did marry her when she was five months pregnant on the other hand, I had known Sebastian for many years; ours was not a brief encounter.

Chapter 3

Andrei's Birth

Towards the end of my pregnancy Sebastian wanted to become a part of it; he attended Lamaze classes and decided to be present during labor.

Furthermore, he arrived at my home on New Years Day to make amends with my family, after all those months, they welcomed him with open arms. Later, Sebastian said he was concerned about the possibility of being unable to reach him if I went into labor. Apparently his mother was aware that the due date was approaching so she began to disconnect the telephone at night, without Sebastian's consent. He later detected this and began to sleep on the sofa in the living room to keep an eye on the telephone in case it rang.

During my last two months, Sebastian began to drive me to and from work. Apart from the emotional stress, I physically felt good during my pregnancy; I never had morning sickness. My feet did begin to swell up towards the end, I also fell at the airport and felt a lot of pressure at the bottom of my belly. After having been checked by the physician, I was no longer able to work until the birth of the baby.

On January 3, 1987, Sebastian and I played dominos until midnight; he left so I could get some rest. At 2:00 am I successfully reached him to tell him that my water had broken and I was having contractions.

Sebastian arrived immediately and we drove together to the hospital as my parents followed. During my labor pains, he kept assuring me of how beautiful it was all going to be with the birth of our baby.

Our baby was born on January 4,1987. Sebastian was the first one to hold him, he brought the baby towards me and I kissed his face. It was a baby boy whom I named Andrei Merlin Romero. He would be the baby who would completely change and bless my whole life and those he came in contact with, my angelic Andrei. When Andrei was brought to me, I felt the touch and warmth of a beautiful innocent baby. I knew I had made the right decision in keeping him and prepared to face whatever would come our way.

Sebastian went to the waiting room and informed my parents, with tears in his eyes, "It was a boy." They all embraced each other and wept. I was put into a recovery room. Minutes later Sebastian came in to see me, kissed me and told me he was so excited with the baby's birth. Then we both began crying.

Soon after, Sebastian approached me in a gentle and loving manner, requesting me to allow his family to meet our baby. He said it was a new beginning with a new life and that we should forgive. I was so happy in giving birth and I indeed loved him, so I permitted his parents to visit. I swallowed my pride and resentment to act as though the nine months of my pregnancy, in which they ignored me, did not bother me. They brought flowers and gifts and were ecstatic about the birth of their first grandson. However, not once did they ever convey any remorse for their treatment of me during my pregnancy.

Driving home from the hospital, Sebastian told me he was going to attempt to be a better person and that we should get married now that the baby was born. He was also very hurt because I would not grant him permission to have the baby bear his last name. I felt differently. Andrei was worthy of having a last name that represented pride and courage. My last name Romero definitely defined that. I explained to Sebastian that, when he actually proved himself to us, the change would be made.

Basically, nothing changed. He continued to be the same, his family never apologized for their behavior towards me and I could no longer act as though it didn't bother me. I was also experiencing post-partum depression. I deceived Sebastian into believing I'd left town but actually kept myself captive in my own home, searching for sanity and tranquillity. He rarely called the house to inquire about the baby and me. After three months of finding peace (and maintaining it to breast-feed) calmly; I resurfaced, calling him to announce I was back in town and that the baby and I were fine. He came over, said that he was not interested in becoming a family and it was over. He did not ask if he could have visits with the baby either. I agreed and told him to leave. I was expecting this and had come to terms with it.

Later I was told he was involved with another woman from the work area. Sebastian transferred on to another department, so I no longer had to work side by side with him when I returned to work. I took six months pregnancy leave; supporting Andrei and myself from my savings. Sebastian was not contributing in any way, shape or form toward Andrei's needs.

The months passed by and Sebastian did not seem to want to get acquainted with his son. We saw Sebastian on three other occasions, the first time was when Andrei was six months. Sebastian's grandmother passed away so I decided to attend the funeral, he and his family were surprised but quite happy to see us there, and to see how beautiful Andrei was becoming. The second occasion was at Andrei's baptism. Father Sean Cronin, whom I had visited upon discovering I was pregnant, baptized him in the same church where I was baptized. The third time, it was at my eldest brother's funeral; Andrei was one month shy of turning a year old. Sebastian briefly attended the funeral. I welcomed him back to the house so that he may spend some time with the baby, he said he would come but to my disappointment he never showed up.

I regularly took Andrei to his "well-baby" check-ups and the pediatrician would always relay his enthusiasm and encouragement of my doing such a wonderful job in raising him. The doctor said Andrei was a healthy baby and was quite amazed that, at nine months old, he already weighed twenty-six pounds. I kept a journal that indicated his first word, first solid meal and first step, and cute things he would do on certain days. I also wrote a long letter to Andrei stating my unconditional love for him and how happy and proud I was to be his mother.

Andrei and I were growing in our relationship. I felt honored to experience the love of a baby, looking up to me, growing bigger and chubbier, saying his first words, taking his first steps, and that beautiful angelic smile he give me. Each and every month I marked his new month of life. His celebration consisted of a cake, reading "Happy 1st Month Andrei", and photos to indicate his growth during that month.

My Angel Andrei

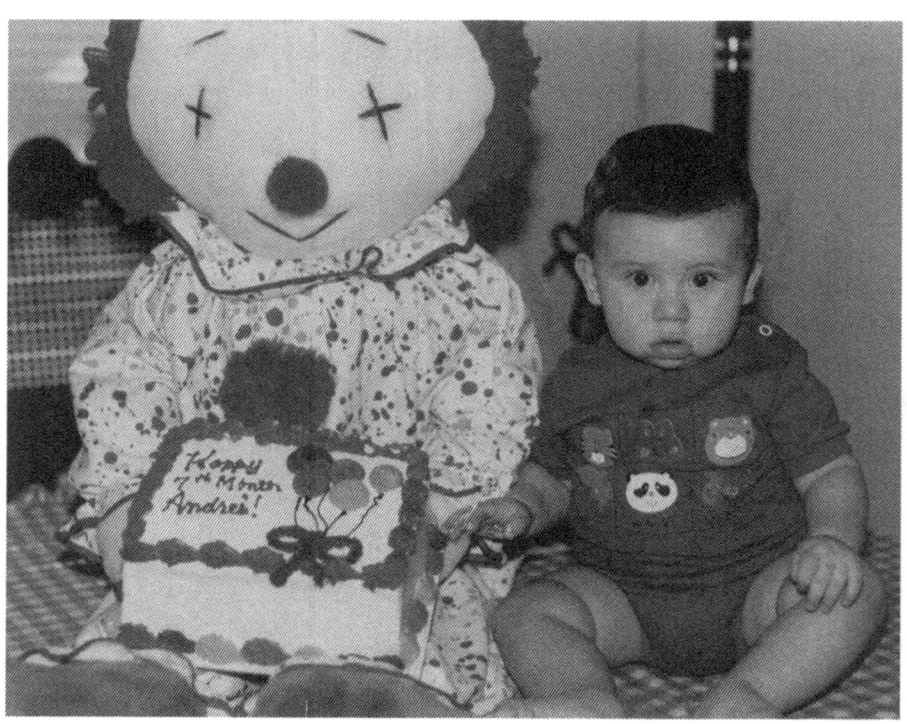

Andrei celebrating seven months of birth

Antoinette Romero

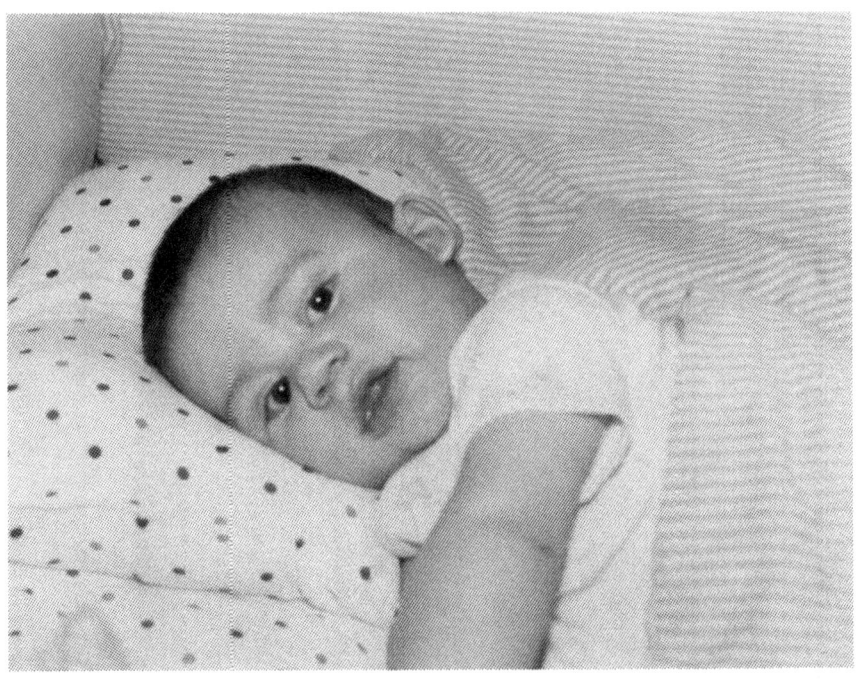

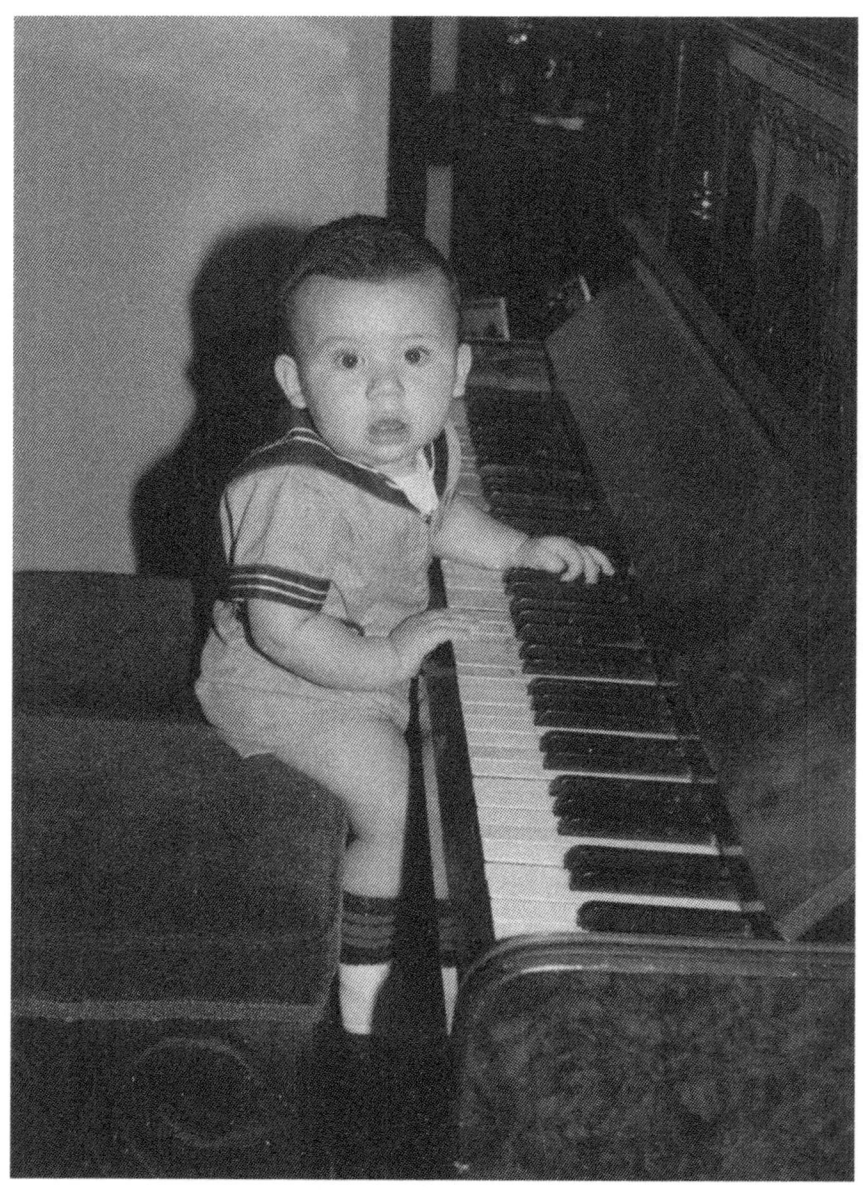

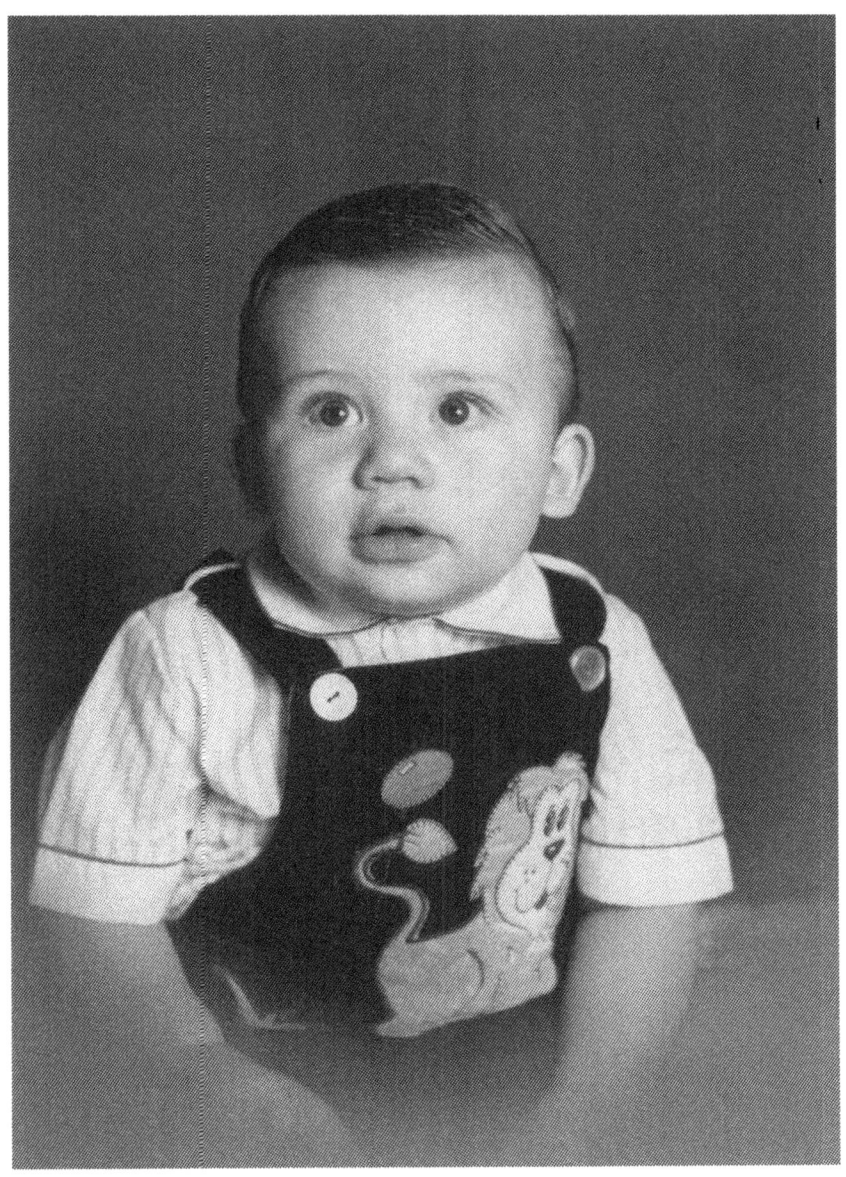

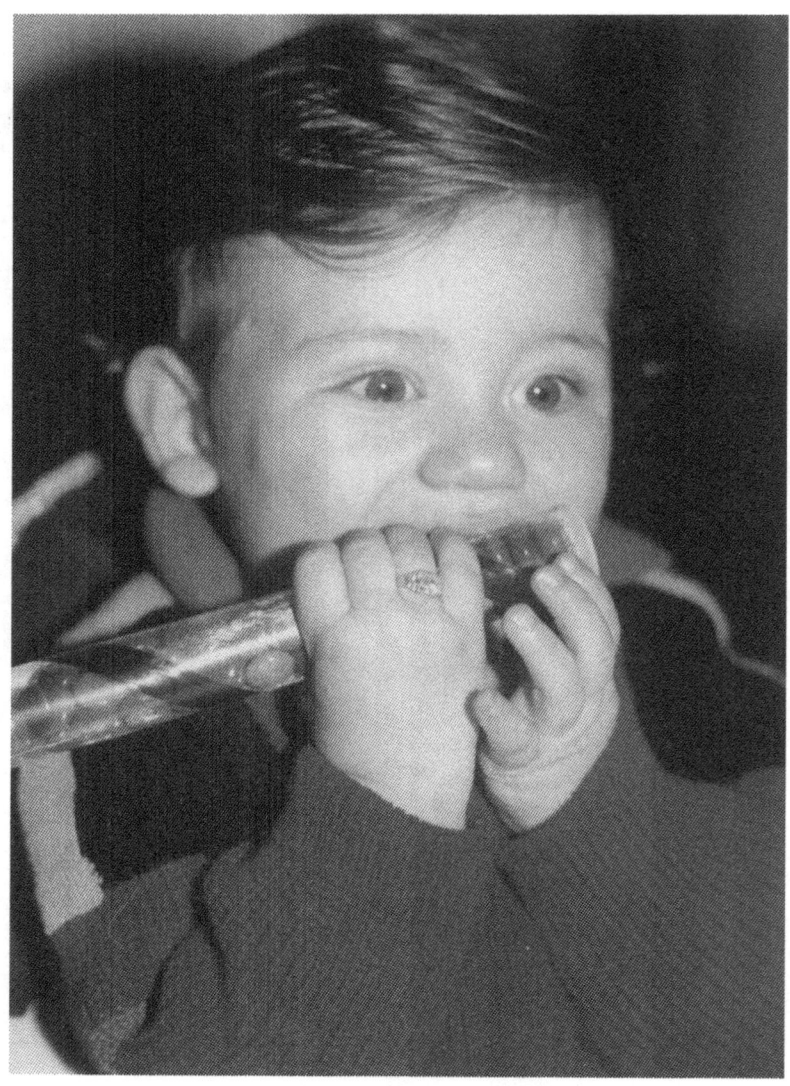

Andrei nine months old

Another year passed, it was 1989 and Andrei was growing quite adorable. I put him into a modeling agency where he was just a ham. He enjoyed having pictures taken of himself and he would pose and have an attitude mixed with a bit of arrogance. Andrei had an incredible personality, always happy, funny and he was a very neat child. He was taught to pick up after himself and he would. We were everything to each other.

Now, when Andrei was two years old, we traveled to Puerto Vallarta, Costa Rica and visited the shrine of the Virgin of Guadeloupe in Mexico City, where I went on a pilgrimage to thank her for the birth of my healthy baby. Andrei had a very kind and generous heart, however, on this trip I had forgotten to pack a single toy for him. When I found a store, I purchased a medium-size plastic car which he loved and carried around the sightseeing areas.

During our daily routine life and even during travels, Andrei always got the attention of people who were always drawn to him in some way. He had these enormous large eyes, kind of hazel with beautiful long eyelashes. His hair was a medium honey brown, complimenting his light-colored skin and there was an aura surrounding him, an unexplainable charisma. He was lovable and very well behaved.

One evening we went out to dinner, and there was a little boy about six years old begging for money. I gave him some money and he took one look at Andrei's car and said to me with the saddest eyes, "Please, can you give me that toy?"

My heart melted but there was not a store in sight where I could purchase one for him. I decided to take a chance with Andrei to see if he might budge and I could take the toy from him to give to the child. I turned to Andrei and said to him in Spanish, "Andrei, this little boy is poor and he has no toys to play with, his mommy has no money to buy him toys, but your mommy can buy you lots of toys and you have many at home. Can you please give this little boy your toy as a gift?"

He listened attentively and, within a second, turned to the boy and rapidly handed him his toy car. I wanted to cry when I witnessed Andrei's generous and understanding response. At such a young age, he was already demonstrating how special he was.

Andrei was well mannered and very disciplined; when we visited friends he would sit next to me politely. For example, one day, we went to my friend Cassandra's house for dinner. Her children ran to the table, but Andrei was missing. Cassandra called him and was amazed to see him putting away the kids' toys in the toy chest before sitting down for dinner.

Andrei was very neat and never wanted his clothes dirty. If he had a T-shirt with any dirty spot, he would immediately want to have it changed. He was finicky in a cute way, almost at times a little 'yuppie.' He enjoyed going shopping with me at grocery stores and malls, and enjoyed riding in the car listening to the music.

One morning I woke up and made a significant decision after much thought and prayer. Before his death, my brother had insisted I request child support from Sebastian, but I was always reluctant. Andrei was growing and soon he would enter pre-school, however, Sebastian had no concern for emotional or financial support. My co-workers told me Sebastian was traveling to Costa Rica, Miami, and Hawaii, and I thought he should contribute to Andrei's upbringing or savings for college.

The previous morning I visited the cemetery and prayed to my brother, Augustine, to guide me in making the right decision and to stand strong. My prayers were answered and I felt confident. I paid a retainer fee to an attorney and took Sebastian to Long Beach Superior Court. I was able to obtain financial support. Surprisingly, Sebastian, requested visitation rights. I was stunned that he wanted to get to know his son.

We were hit with another loss eight months after Augustine died. My brother, Gerald, was suddenly taken to the hospital for abdominal pains; he died suddenly three days later. All of us including Andrei, were confused by this trauma. My parents signed consent forms for an autopsy but California law only allows "next of kin" to grant permission. His daughters were too young and their mother didn't grant this for her own reasons.

Sebastian began visiting with Andrei on a weekly basis for two hours. My sister or mother had to be present because Andrei who was two years of age did not feel comfortable with him and he would cry since Sebastian was a stranger to him.

I would go to work and allow them to become acquainted with each other. Sebastian later confessed that he was quite surprised when he saw Andrei, he never imagined him to be so grown up and speaking words. The weeks went by and Sebastian was now permitted to have Andrei for an entire afternoon.

One day we were on the sidewalk waiting for Sebastian to pick up Andrei when I saw Sebastian's car approaching. I turned to Andrei and said, "Look, there's Papa."

From that day on Andrei called Sebastian, "Papa" as if he felt he was granted permission from his mother to call this man by his actual relationship with him. For a short period of time, they spent afternoons together, and Sebastian's parents were also able get acquainted with their grandson.

Sebastian once again was beginning to slack off. On many visiting days, if he did not show up late, he would not show up at all. I was getting angry because it would hurt me to see Andrei looking out the window waiting for his father.

On several occasions, I told Mrs. Carrillo, Sebastian's mother, that it was not fair to Andrei to be put through this. She would agree and say she would have a talk with her son. I felt I had to struggle with his flakiness once again, and this time it was not about me but the person I most loved. I would not allow Andrei to get hurt, I needed to protect him.

When Sebastian was spending some more time with Andrei, we began to have more rapport with each other. When he would come to pick up Andrei, he sometimes would not leave immediately but try to stay and talk to me, inquiring if I was dating or if I had any feelings for him. I realized I still felt something for him. I became involved with him once again, probably fantasizing we would become a family. It ended when Lourdes told me Sebastian was still seeing his old girlfriend but she had been away during the time I began to get involved with him. I was hurt but would not believe it completely until I confronted him, I called his house and a woman answered the telephone. When Sebastian took the telephone from her, I yelled and cried, telling him he did not have to do this to me. It was the ending of what I believed to be the beginning.

I continued hearing about Sebastian dating women and even saw him one day at the mall buying Andrei's Christmas gift with one of his female friends. I was with my sister, Linda, and Andrei, buying chocolate milk for his bottle, when we saw each other and he became extremely nervous. I guess he believed I would make a scene. I smiled and greeted them both and walked away with the stroller.

The following morning he came to visit with Andrei and I did not mention a word until he felt the need to explain. I said I did not need or want to know anything. I lied and said I just wanted him to be happy! Although I was hurt and angry, I did not let him know. Why was he coming back into our life to disrupt and confuse us?

Once again, Sebastian vanished from Andrei's life and mine and his responsibility as a decent father. It was not always easy because I was still deeply in love with Sebastian. I knew that I needed to move on and having Andrei by my side gave me the strength to struggle with my emotions and insecurities. I was fine raising Andrei on my own and I was very happy being a mother, he was a blessing. Our relationship was magnificent.

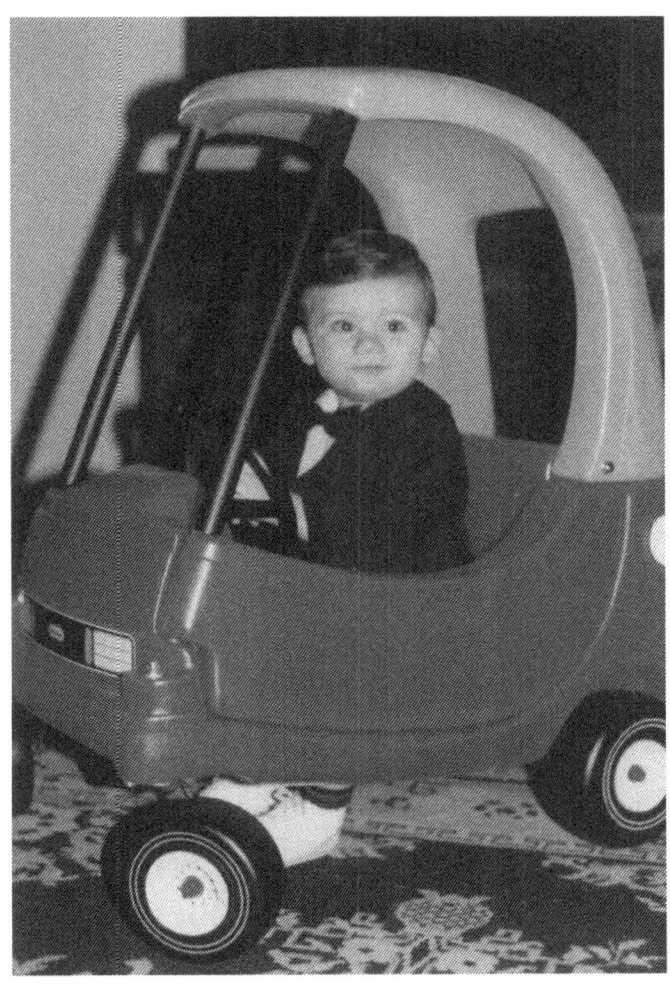

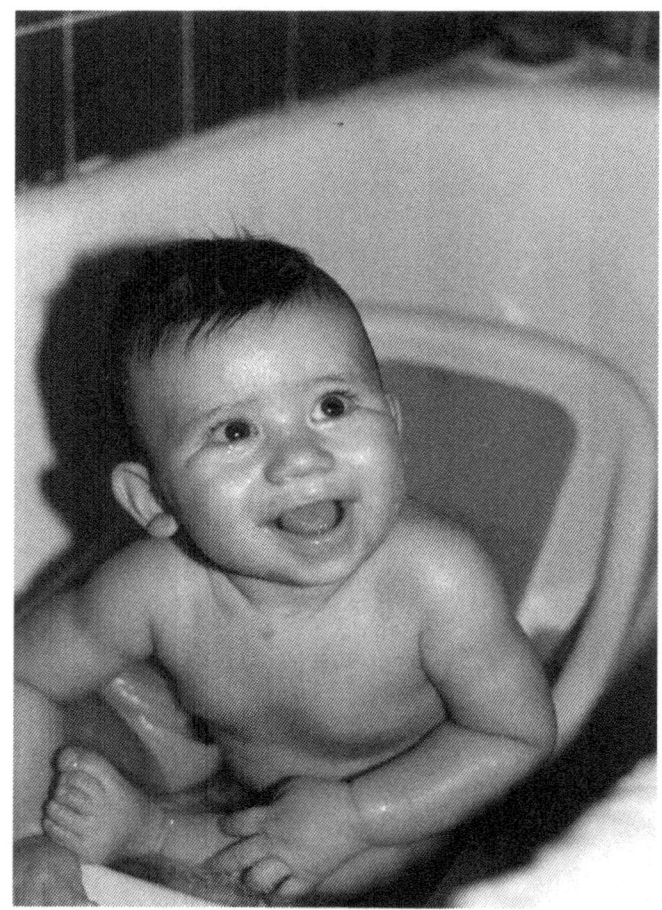

Andrei in the bathtub

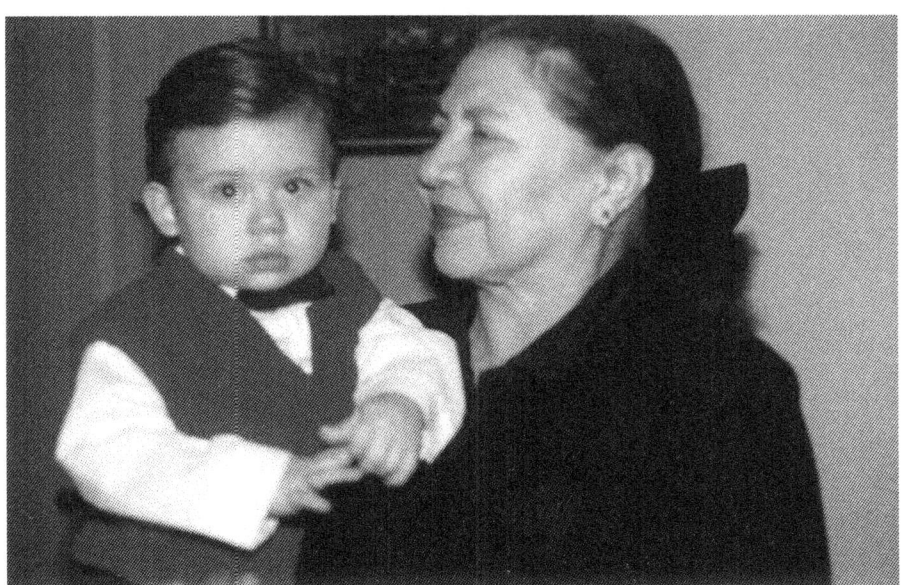

Andrei being held by Grandma

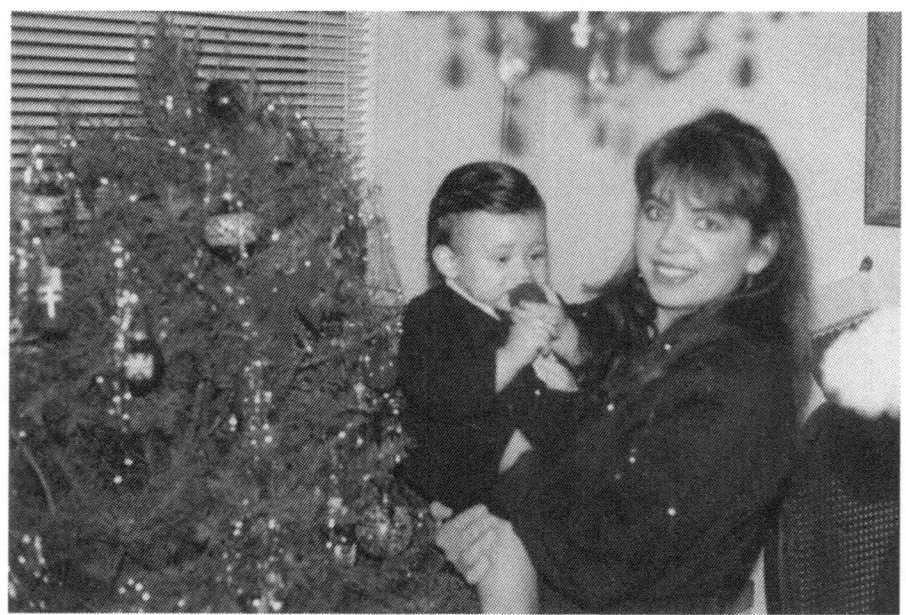

Andrei and Mommy celebrating his first Christmas

Chapter 4
First Signs and Diagnosis

It was June of 1989 and suddenly Andrei began to have frequent ear infections and the doctor advised us that he would have to perform surgery to insert "ear tubes" for the problem. It was a simple procedure but anesthesia would be administered. I was so afraid and concerned about any danger his life might be in, but the physician assured me it was not dangerous. It was an outpatient procedure and I could take him home the same day. I was so nervous during surgery and unaware of what would lie ahead for Andrei and me. My parents accompanied me and all went well. We were relieved.

Then Andrei's personality began to change drastically and I could not comprehend what the problem was. He was two-and-a-half years old and was becoming very irritable; I thought maybe it was "the terrible two's" syndrome. I took some vacation time from work and arranged to take Andrei to his pediatrician for an examination. The doctor's concern was the weight loss; I explained how Andrei had not been himself lately. The doctor began to see him almost on a daily basis, and every day there was at least an ounce of weight loss, which was peculiar.

We were also dispatched after every visit to the Little Company of Mary Hospital to have blood work done. Andrei's reaction was astounding. When we first entered the parking lot of the hospital he would cry and say "No, Mommy" and didn't want to leave the car. He was aware of the procedure.

I would carry him into the hospital but, once he was laid on the bed and his arm was extended to draw the blood, he would bravely turn his head away to the other side and cooperate with the procedure. He was very courageous young child aware he had to go through this.

The only physical evidence which resulted from the tests was a high sed (sedimentation) rate, which indicated there was something wrong, but not specific in which area. I continued to take Andrei, five days a week and the same procedures were done over and over. He also had many ear infections and the doctor found a growth on his tongue and mouth called thrush. It was a sort of fungus. The doctor believed this possibly was the reason for Andrei not having an appetite due to the discomfort inside his mouth. I also took Andrei to a "Natural Healer." It was a bit out of the ordinary, but I was desperate and tried everything I possibly could.

In addition, many other tests were performed on him, such as an ultrasound on his abdomen, lupus, AIDS, I noticed he was deteriorating everyday. I took him to the emergency room at Cedars-Sinai Hospital where a pediatric physician examined and observed him. Andrei cried and screamed because he was frightened and in pain wherever his problem was. She informed me at that time she believed there was nothing physically wrong with him but she did diagnose an "emotional" problem, *"How ridiculous,"* I thought to myself. She was the resident physician and it appeared she did not have much experience in the field, obviously assuming a psychological problem without running any tests. Her judgment did not seem accurate to me and I was unsatisfied with her diagnosis.

Days later, I took Andrei to the Torrance Memorial Hospital emergency room; where a doctor on call examined him. X-rays oddly demonstrated an accumulation of stool in his stomach. The doctor's diagnosis said that Andrei was emotionally disturbed and he was refraining from bowel movements to prove to me he was in control of his own body. The doctor also insinuated many times that I was an overprotective mother and there was nothing medically wrong with my son.

So a few days later, I took Andrei to the Long Beach Memorial Hospital emergency room where the doctors also saw the bowel accumulation in his stomach and directed me to a Pediatric specialist. I took him to a specialist and he said, "We are looking into a dark room where we do not know what we are looking for."

He also said the illness could be chronic or terminal, I was directed to come back for further tests.

I then decided to return to his regular pediatrician, until his next appointment. I wanted to explain to her about the doctors I had been visiting. She sent me to a family therapist, also believing what her colleague said was an emotional problem for the moment until the results of other tests returned. I went on to do everything in my power to look for answers. I entered the therapist's room as suggested with Andrei, Mom and Dad. We had a full hour session and she did not presume there was a psychological problem.

Although his father never played a significant role in his life, Andrei was not emotionally affected. His role models were my parents and myself and we were raising him with tender love and care. It is important to have a father around but I could not force Sebastian to be someone he did not want to be; fatherhood is something that should be felt naturally and instinctively.

By now, a two months had passed. I continued with my persistence with Andrei's doctor and she continued to run tests. Finally, she told me all the tests she could possibly order had been performed and the only final tests to do were a CT Scan and an MRI. These two tests were scheduled for the following days.

I went to Sunday mass with Andrei and my mother. As we were leaving, my grammar school teacher, Sister Angela, was also walking out. We approached each other and embraced, at this moment Andrei was swinging on the pole of the ramp outside the church. I pointed to him and said to Sister Angela, "Look, that little boy is my son, Andrei."

She grabbed him and hugged him; I then told her about his undiagnosed illness. We exchanged telephone numbers and she said she would keep him in her prayers and for me to contact her once I had some news.

Sebastian reappeared soon after I called to tell him I was taking the baby to the doctors because I suspected something was wrong. He was very uncooperative in the beginning, also suggested I was overprotective and there was most likely nothing wrong with him. When I asked him for help, he took off for Costa Rica for a school reunion and returned four days later.

I was very angry with him. His mother called and said she wanted to accompany me to those particular tests. I guess she was trying to stand in for Sebastian because I would not talk to him after he returned. Mrs. Carrillo and my mother accompanied us to the hospital for the tests. My mother was a significant support, she constantly advised me to make more appointments for further evaluations. She insisted that I go to the emergency rooms at the hospitals for immediate attention and she went with me to all the appointments.

To keep Andrei from being frightened by the large machines, I pleaded to be allowed to stand by his side during the MRI test. I would tell him he was in an airplane and was going to fly because he loved airplanes since he knew I worked at the airport.

We finished the test procedure and the technician looked extremely concerned; we were immediately taken to the CT-Scan room. Once again, the new technician also looked concerned; he instructed me to go directly to the doctor's office. As I carried Andrei through the hallway to get to my mother and Mrs. Carrillo, I began to cry. I was frightened; I had a hunch something was wrong. Andrei was asleep due to the sedative they had given him during the tests so he was not able to see how upset I was.

When I approached my mother and Mrs. Carrillo, I signed to Mrs. Carrillo not to say anything to my mother that I was crying. I told them the results were complete and the doctor on call wanted me to go to his office immediately; it was just down the street, so we arrived quickly. I told them to stay in the car since Andrei was still asleep. When I got to the doctor's office and gave my name, the nurse asked who was with me. I said my mother was in the car since my son was asleep and she said I had to bring in the people who were accompanying me. When I was returning to the car all sorts of things were going through my mind, but I told both mothers they needed to get out of the car and go in with me. I carried Andrei who was completely sedated. When we walked in, we were taken to a private room; I was nervous and shaking all over. I never could have imagined what sort of news the doctor was going to give me.

The doctor walked in, sat down and first confided that he needed to apologize to me. Because of my persistence they were able to diagnose Andrei. Then he said, "I am very sorry, Antoinette, but we discovered a brain tumor in Andrei."

I remember screaming and crying. His nurse came in the room and also began crying and offered me water. Mrs. Carrillo grabbed Andrei away from my arms so that my mother could reach out to me, and we both cried and embraced each other.

The doctor gave me the name of a pediatric neurosurgeon in Long Beach, Dr. Stevenson; he also gave me his home phone number and told me to call at any time. He was just trying to feel better since he was so rude and cruel with me during the emergency room visits. As we were driving back home, all of us in shock, I pleaded with Mrs. Carrillo to speak to her son and help him get his act together, because this was the time Andrei was going to need his father around.

When we arrived home, I went to lay Andrei on the bed and laid down beside him. I held him in my arms and cried myself to sleep, but Andrei still had the effect of the sedation. Soon after, Sebastian arrived at my house and sat beside us. He woke me up and apologized for not believing in me when I kept telling him there was something wrong with the baby. The physician said they had never had any cases like Andrei's; they were definitely going to change their methods and begin to take mothers quite seriously when they insisted something was not right with their child.

Chapter 5

Confusion and Choosing a Surgeon

We were referred to a specialist and the following day we went to see the pediatric neurosurgeon in Long Beach, who told us of the possibility of the tumor being a Chordoma. It is a very rare, malignant tumor, located in the back of the brain by the cerebellum. Andrei was hospitalized that day and many tests were done; the same ones and new ones. Andrei was so frightened by the hospital that he wouldn't even sleep in his bed. He wanted me to hold him in my arms, so we would sit on a recliner chair and sleep there together holding on to each other. If I needed to go to the restroom, eat or go to the house to shower and change, I could only do it if my mother took my place, also holding him. My family was incredibly supportive and loving, they were my sole support and I could not have gotten through this without them.

Five days went by and nothing was being done. My sister, Linda, and I accidentally ran into the doctor while going to donate blood for Andrei's surgery. I questioned the doctor on what was going on because he had stopped coming in to examine the baby and we were confused. I insisted he come in and be honest with us so the following day he met with me, Sebastian, my parents and sister. He had a skeleton of a head to show us where the tumor was. He explained the seriousness of the problem to us and told Sebastian and myself that these situations either "make or break us."

I guess he believed we were married and said many men run because they cannot handle such major stress. Ironically, it made sense later. The doctor informed us how he was going to perform the surgery, he wanted to go through Andrei's jaw to try to get to the tumor. We were all scared and confused but were going to allow this surgery because we wanted to have confidence in this doctor.

The surgery was one day away and the doctor had still not come in to speak to us. I told the nurse I needed to see the doctor. At that time, they told me the surgery was canceled with no explanation and no doctor to be seen for the next three days. We were stunned!

After an entire week at the hospital they discharged us without any explanation. The nurse told me to call the doctor's office in a few days to reschedule a surgery date. When I asked her what should I do if something went wrong at home, she said "call 911."

I was appalled and could not comprehend why they were trying to get rid of us. By mere coincidence, in the hall, my sister had run into the doctor again, and it seemed he was afraid to perform the surgery or was uncertain since these types of surgeries are difficult in a rare tumor case.

As soon as we arrived home, my sister, Linda, began to look for telephone numbers of pediatric neurosurgeons. One doctor from UCLA, Dr. Palmer, was said to be one of the best, however, he was in India when I tried to set up an appointment. We went to see a doctor from Los Angeles Children's Hospital, Dr. Travis, who informed us if he performed the surgery the tumor would eventually grow back, and that would cause his death. I was in shock; this was the first time someone told me Andrei could die from his tumor. I obviously became angry and did not want this doctor to be the one to perform the surgery, since I perceived him to be negative; I did not like what I was hearing.

Many days went by and Linda had contacted pediatric neurosurgeons at the Mayo Clinic and at Cedars Sinai Hospital. We went to see Dr. Mitchell Graine from Cedars Sinai; the first impression I got was a positive one. He looked assertive and intelligent and, most of all, when he spoke to us, he gave us the response we were searching for. He said he had already performed this same surgery on a young seven year old Persian boy who had had good results with surgery, with chemotherapy and radiation. The child was still alive and doing well. The doctor did not seem insecure in performing the surgery and his confidence made us feel secure and trusting that Andrei would be in good hands.

The doctor allowed us to take some time to think about him and to consider other physicians. By the next day we had made our decision, it would be Dr. Graine. I called the doctor and told him our decision was with him.

Andrei was going to be admitted to the hospital the next day, September 25, 1989. As we were getting ready to leave, Andrei ran back to the house where my mother was at the door giving us her blessing. Andrei approached her and whispered through the screen door, "Nana, are you coming with us?" and Mother told him she would arrive later. My poor child had no idea what was going to be occurring within the next few days.

Before he was admitted, Sebastian and I took him to a pet shop to play with some puppies because he kept saying he wanted a little doggie. The store allowed him to carry and play with puppies and then I told Andrei, "As soon as you get well, we will come to the store and Mommy will buy you a doggie."

Andrei would become happy, smile and reply, "OK, but only a little one, Mommy," making a gesture with his fingers for 'little.'

My Angel Andrei

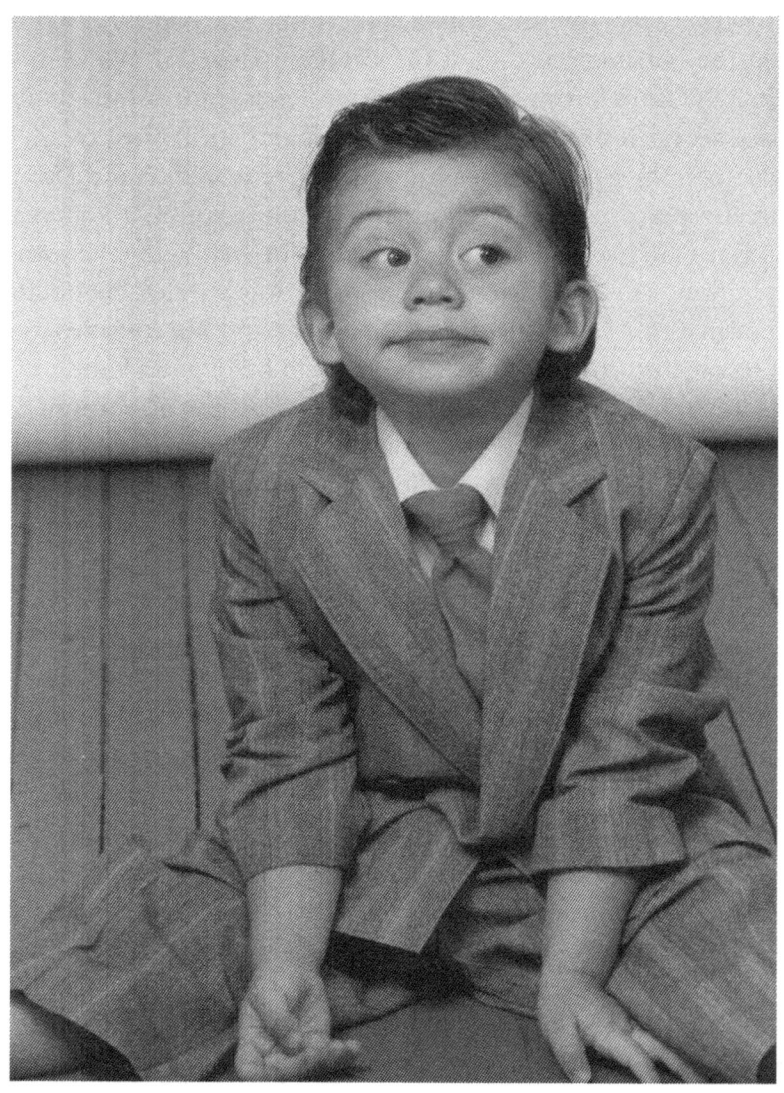

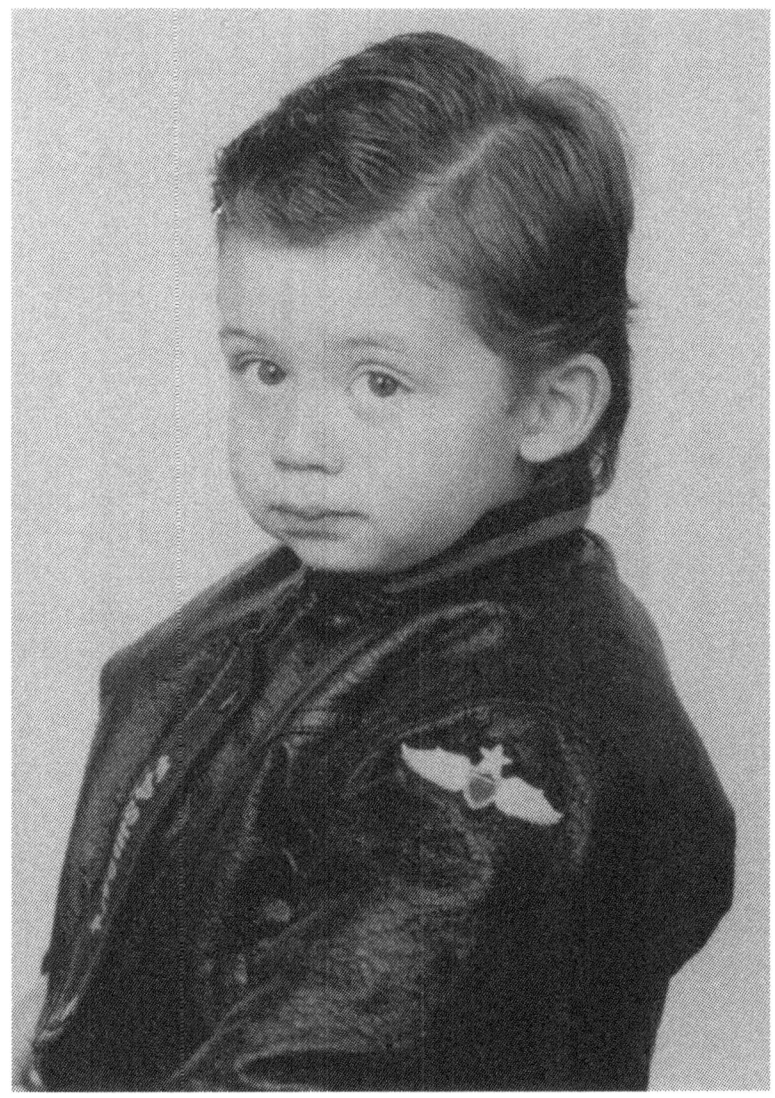

Chapter 6

The Surgery and Post-Op

We arrived at the hospital in the evening; Sebastian and I slept in the room with the baby. It was a difficult night because Andrei was afraid and nurses and the doctor on call kept coming into the room checking up on him, asking many questions.

The following morning he was sent to have new tests performed (CT scan and MRI); I waited outside as they instructed me. The doctor arrived a few minutes later and told me it would be awhile. During the wait, Andrei walked out to the hall and put his head against the wall, angrily saying he wanted to leave. I ran after him and persuaded him to go back to the waiting area with me. I never imagined it would be the last time I would see him walk or run again. He was taken in for the tests and I was not permitted to go in with him; I waited anxiously outside in the waiting room pacing the floor and praying.

When Andrei was brought out, I was stunned. My baby was not the same, he was intubated with all these tubes through his mouth. I began to cry once I saw him. The doctor explained Andrei's true vocal cords did not abduct and he had no gag reflex which is why he had to undergo intubation. I called home so that my parents could come and stay with me; we all tried to be very strong so that we would not frighten Andrei.

Sebastian arrived later on that evening. It was supposed to be a simple procedure and nobody expected this to occur.

Dr. Graine told me the surgery would be September 28. He sat with us and explained his procedure for the surgery; he would go through the back of the skull by the cerebellum. He was quite frank and did specify Andrei could possibly not make it through this long surgery. This was a very difficult decision, but I knew it had to be done and I knew I had to trust in God. This was definitely a testing time for me and my religion. I consider myself strong in my faith, although this was something too complex to understand. I questioned God why a child has to suffer?

Andrei went into surgery at about 6.00 a.m. my family and friends were beside me, and also Sebastian was there with his family. I made sure Father Sean Cronin gave the baby his blessing and we all prayed over him so that he would make it through surgery. Surgery lasted nine long hours, in the first four hours, the doctor called up to the waiting room to update us about the surgery's progress. Dr. Graine told us he had already opened up the area and was about to go in to retrieve the tumor.

Those were the longest hours I had ever experienced of frustration and despair. I was extremely nervous. After a long wait, the doctor came out in his scrubs to notify us Andrei had made it through the surgery. However, he was unable to retract all the tumor because it was hard as wood and there were some important nerves surrounding the tumor. He suggested that, maybe with chemotherapy and radiation treatments, they would be able to get the rest of the remaining tumor or at least shrink the size of it.

After an hour, Andrei came out of the recovery room. My baby looked so different, it was a frightening sight. His head had been shaved, and his beautiful honey brown hair was gone. His little head was wrapped in gauze and he was on a respirator, and all kinds of tubes covered him and his crib. He was still under the effect of the anesthesia; hours went by and he wouldn't wake up. I slept next to Andrei's crib in a chair. When I stood next to him, trying to comprehend why this was happening to us, I began to cry as I looked at Andrei's little body connected to a respirator to help him breathe. I was inconsolable. When Andrei opened his eyes, he looked at me, briefly smiled, puckered his lips and blew a kiss at me. I was so thrilled, I took this as a message from my little angel telling me, "Mommy, it's going to be OK, hang in there."

From that day forward, I became energized as though I was injected with some boost of positive thinking. I made a promise to myself at that moment I was not going to give up on Andrei or feel sorry for what we were going through. I began to read a book about being well and thinking positive. It's described how, if you believe in something with all your heart, you convince yourself you are going to become well. With positive thinking and living your life with that attitude, one's life can be extended or cured with the positive waves you feed your brain.

I knew if I began to act on this and to feel as though I was the one diagnosed with a terminal illness, Andrei would feed on this. Andrei would see me always positive, happy and full of positive energy when I was around him continuously. I made sure I looked well groomed as he was also accustomed to seeing me that way. If you try to look good, you tend to feel a bit better.

I also discovered a new form of communication for Andrei and myself. I taught him to flutter his eyelashes or blow a kiss for "Yes" and frown for "No," as we were unable to talk.

Soon after his surgery, we began to notice Andrei did not have any lower body movement, nor any in his right arm. Dr. Graine would come in and poke a needle into Andrei's foot and nothing would happen; he could not feel a thing. Apparently some nerves became damaged after the surgery, causing paralysis.

As the days went by, things got worse. I was notified that Andrei could not have a foreign object in his body for long and they would have to insert a trachea tube to help his breathing. Then Andrei began to experience epileptic attacks and new medication had to be added to his regular doses. With great effort in the months to come, he did learn to talk again. He had another surgery to insert a gastrostomy tube in which he received daily feeding. A Brovia Catheter (central line) was connected to his small chest so that chemotherapy could be administered and blood drawn.

In essence, everything was changing; my baby was no longer permitted to be a baby. For example, Andrei's nickname for his bottle was 'Bu.' He truly enjoyed it. I hadn't been able to wean him off it and now he was unable to drink from it. He wouldn't take a nap nor go to sleep without it so I knew that he wanted his Bu. I took a bottle from the unit, filled it with milk and put it towards his mouth. Although he couldn't suck on it, he was content and satisfied with having the bottle in his mouth and able to feel it.

The doctors had apparently told my family that Andrei had only two months to live; they all kept it from me for fear of what I might do to myself. I had been telling my mother that, if Andrei died, I was going with him. I could not bear the thought of losing him; since Andrei was my whole life, I felt it would be useless to live without him. I honestly contemplated suicide and would think of ways to try to take my life if Andrei should die. When my mother heard me talk this way, she contacted Sister Angela, to give me a spiritual uplift. My family feared that I would not be able to cope with losing my beautiful baby.

After a few weeks, Dr. Hensley, the oncologist, walked in one day to discuss chemotherapy for Andrei. I approached her and, with tears in my eyes, pleaded with her to tell me what she believed were Andrei's chances. I told her I had every right to know. At her office, she sat me down to explain the seriousness of Andrei's health and that he may have only a month or so to live.

I looked into her eyes and told her Andrei was going to make it. I said I was going to help him fight the odds. She looked at me as she had probably looked at many other parents to whom she'd had to break this devastating news. I walked away and ran into Sebastian whose part in this situation was unthinkable. I believe now he was probably as frightened as I was, however, his way of dealing with it was very selfish and cowardly. He was not taking any responsibility for any decisions; it was all up to me. I felt frustrated and resentful.

On the day of the surgery for the G-Tube (gastrostomy tube), Sebastian told me he was leaving the hospital. I asked him how could he leave knowing his son was going to have surgery and have a tube inserted into his stomach.

He said, "Oh it's only an hour-and-a-half surgery, he will be fine."

I exploded, saying, "You can't leave, why are you doing this to us?"

I began to cry hysterically. My mother was with me then and she turned to me, saying, "Why are you begging him to stay, where is your dignity."

I reacted to her words, composed myself and let him go.

I would have to say that literally I let him go. What I mean by this is that I made the decision not to pursue Sebastian anymore or try to have him be around us, supporting us through this awful crisis. I had been trying to persuade Sebastian that he needed to be around to help me make the decisions on the healthcare or treatments for Andrei. I guess I thought I needed emotional support from the man I truly loved, but actually I needed sanity and he was not allowing me to have that. His presence was only causing me to be and act dysfunctional. I was concentrating more on Sebastian's behavior instead of on my son who needed my total attention and care.

Furthermore, Sebastian parents demanded him to go home for the weekend to house sit, because the house could not be left alone, in case of a burglary. They were leaving to San Diego for the weekend to visit with their daughter. I went insane, I packed Sebastian's belongings and simply requested he leaves and never come back. I also insinuated to Sebastian I did not want to see his hypocritical parents; they only made me miserable and were not assisting me in any way.

I honestly questioned the purpose of their visits, especially when a longtime friend of theirs confessed to me that a well-known priest from

Costa Rica was traveling through Los Angeles to Taipei, and she was going to bring him to the hospital to pray over Andrei. However, his visit would be brief since he did not have much time between planes. Apparently, Sebastian's parents were aware of the time restriction and pleaded with their friend, Elvira, for the priest to visit their son first.

Regardless of their reasons, it was selfish not to think of Andrei who was fighting for his life. I was disgusted with them and felt they were only a burden. I could not deal with it anymore and I was extremely depressed and stressed out.

Instead of understanding my anxieties and nervousness, they criticized it, made no effort to sit down and talk to me about how we should all try to get along nor did they demonstrate any compassion. What they did do was react with condescension and resentment towards me. I did not deserve to be treated this way; I was a mother trying to understand my child's struggle for life.

I wanted them to say that it mattered to be around Andrei but I guess their dislike towards me and pride meant more to them. I never saw them again; they never called or attempted any communication. Sebastian also swayed towards their opinion and his conduct demonstrated it over time.

From that day forward, I analyzed my behavior and how I was putting too much effort on Sebastian. Weekends would come and he would disappear; then he would tell me how tired he was from working. I later would discover from my friends how they would run into him at a party, but would keep it from me for fear of getting me more upset and depressed with my whole ordeal. One night they ran into him at a foreign consulate party and he was really enjoying himself; how could he when I was at the hospital with his son in the intensive care unit fighting for Andrei's life!

After the G-Tube surgery, Andrei had a vein that was not cauterized properly so he began bleeding to the extent of losing a pint of blood total and he needed a transfusion once in the morning. Throughout the night, resident doctors and surgeons kept coming in to see Andrei. But nothing was done about his bleeding, all they would do is wrap gauze around his torso; it was very messy and bloody. The doctors asked if I preferred to leave so that I would not become sick; I had to be brave, say no and stay so that Andrei would not be afraid. I told Andrei to look away and just look into my face while they healed his owie. Andrei appeared very afraid, but he was obedient and never looked down to see what the doctors were doing. At one point, three doctors were there at once.

It was difficult for me because I have always had a weak stomach, but I somehow got the strength to stay beside him. During all this time, the nurses on call were trying to reach Sebastian who was nowhere to be found. His mother would answer the phone and not even try to inquire if this had to do with something serious about Andrei. Sebastian finally called the next morning at 11:00 a.m., apparently the time he arrived home. I was so furious I could not take his call.

About 7:00 a.m. Andrei went back into surgery to have the vein cauterized; when he came out, his entire little chest was stapled down to close the opening across it. The appalling thing was that the doctors did not seem to worry until Andrei had lost a lot of blood. The doctors came in after his surgery and I told them exactly how I felt. At this point I was extremely upset and emotionally exhausted from staying up all night so maybe it was understandable why I reacted this way.

I told them I was angry, and Andrei has been through enough and does not need this kind of negligence to occur. The doctors were apologetic and sympathetic to my words.

Unfortunately, I encountered many unpleasant situations. One physician bluntly came out and told me that Andrei was not going to make it and my hopes would not become a reality.

How dare he? I thought to myself. Then I told him he was wrong, I told him Andrei was going to be one of those rare cases that was going to be a miracle, we were fighters and were not going to give up on each other. One of the nurses told me later he had lost a son to AIDS a month prior; I believe he was just bitter and angry and probably did not mean any of it.

Another incident occurred when Andrei was going to be fitted for orthopedic braces for the soles of his feet. Since he was paralyzed, the bottoms of his feet needed to become upright because they were losing their form. The doctor who specialized in making the foot brace forms turned to me and asked why was this being done if he was a terminal patient. I was stunned and insisted I was not leaving until he made these braces for my child.

I had been experiencing so much stress and, after truly reviewing my situation, I decided to give up on Sebastian. I wanted to value myself with a little more dignity and respect. Sebastian's last visit with Andrei was that day of his G-Tube surgery and, when he left, he never came back. I no longer called him or made any efforts to contact him nor did he try to contact me. I think the day of Andrei's incident Sebastian really got scared, so much so that his way of dealing with this was through denial and staying away from reality. He also, did not want to deal with my "nagging" about his inconsistency and coldness. I, on the other hand, became a very strong woman and began to feel and act positive around Andrei. I honestly believed in my heart he would survive and pull through this. The oncologist came in to discuss his chemotherapy and the radiologist came to discuss his radiation treatments.

After the biopsy, the tumor was sent to a pathologist in Boston who finally diagnosed it as a very rare tumor named Chordoma. It is so rare that no protocol exists to treat it. The few patients who have been diagnosed have been primarily adults, it rarely occurs in children. The doctors combined their knowledge, experience and wisdom to use the treatments they thought to be most suitable. Andrei was administered a strong dosage of chemo for a period of five days every three weeks. To the amazement of doctors and nurses, Andrei was not becoming sick with nausea. Although I was being told the chemo was very strong, they could not believe how well his body was responding to the chemotherapy. There were other bright spots, too.

One day for example, I brought in his cassette player with one of his favorite songs that had an upbeat rhythm, the title of the song is "You're My One and Only." When Andrei would ride in the car, he would slip the cassette in right away to hear this song. We played it loudly next to his ears and I told him to try to move to the music. All of a sudden, he tilted his head to the right moving to the beat of the music. I was so delighted I began going around the hospital unit telling everyone of Andrei's progress.

I went with Andrei everywhere I was allowed to accompany him. During his radiation treatments, when he was asked to remain totally immobile as he received radiation, it was my voice that was "piped" into the treatment area to calm his anxieties and dry his tears. He wore a customized head set for the radiation treatments.

On one occasion, just before we went in for one of Andrei's treatments, we ran into Sammy Davis Jr. who was being treated for his own cancer. He looked at Andrei as though feeling great compassion for him. I guess it probably made him not feel so bad for himself seeing a small child going through the same process of treatments as he was. We looked at each other and smiled warmly.

Before Andrei's treatments, doctors discussed a possibility of his being a candidate at Stanford Medical Center for a new procedure which involved a high dose of radiation with a special beam. The outcomes were said to be excellent. However, Stanford doctors returned its answer saying could not take him in because they did not believe he was a valid candidate for success, since he was paralyzed and his prognosis did not look well after his surgery.

I was devastated once again, having to hear something negative, but I did not allow it to block my attitude, spirituality and faith. Dr. Matrix, the doctor in charge of his radiation treatments, was intrigued with my personal life and began to try to discuss with me why I was not married to Sebastian. It appeared as if word had spread around the hospital unit and the personnel were somehow also intrigued.

Subsequently, the nurses called Sebastian, "Mr. Romero." Sebastian pleaded with me not to say anything since he was embarrassed if they knew otherwise. I was disappointed at the attitude and the gossip that circulated at the hospital regarding the fact that I was not married to Sebastian. Some doctors were very kind and considerate, as well as many of the nurses. Since I was sleeping on a daily basis in a chair next to Andrei's crib, a certain resident doctor would come beside me and put a blanket over me. Many of them sympathized with me, particularly because they acknowledged the love Andrei and I shared for each other. Many of the children who were hospitalized did not have their mothers or fathers by their bedside twenty -four hours a day. Whatever the reasons, these children were alone most of the time.

One day, I experienced a lapse of weakness and decided to call Sebastian. When I called, his telephone number was disconnected and the operator had no forwarding number. I was overcome, unable to comprehend how he had never called me to give me his new number. I thought, "What if Andrei became seriously ill, or died? How was I going to contact him? "

The following day when I went to his house, a stranger opened the door. I asked to see Sebastian, he informed me he and his wife were the new owners of the house and Sebastian no longer lived there. I felt a sharp pain in my chest, walked away, got in my car and cried during the drive home. I couldn't believe my ears, I was dazed and saddened by this news. I then called Sebastian at work; they told me he had taken a few days off.

It was about a week later when I was able to locate him at work. I began crying when I heard his voice and said, "I cannot believe you moved and did not even advise me of your new telephone number. How am I to contact you if something happens to Andrei, doesn't he signify anything to you?"

He was silent and told me he was going to call me that night to talk. Later that evening, he called the Intensive Care Unit and gave me his new number so that I could call him collect from a public phone in order to speak in private. I called him and we talked extensively. What I perceived from the conversation was that his parents did not want me to know his whereabouts and they were prohibiting him from giving the number to me. He said he was repentant once again for his behavior and soon he would contact me.

I later spoke to Sebastian's older brother Gary, the one person I can honestly say was kind and caring and, the only family member who supported me. I called him to discuss Sebastian's behavior. He told me he was aware of his parents' meddling and did not approve of their behavior and particularly how they succeeded in controlling him. He did say he believed Sebastian loved Andrei and me, however, because of their parent's involvement, Sebastian was incapable to stand up for what he really wanted to do. I thanked Gary for all his support.

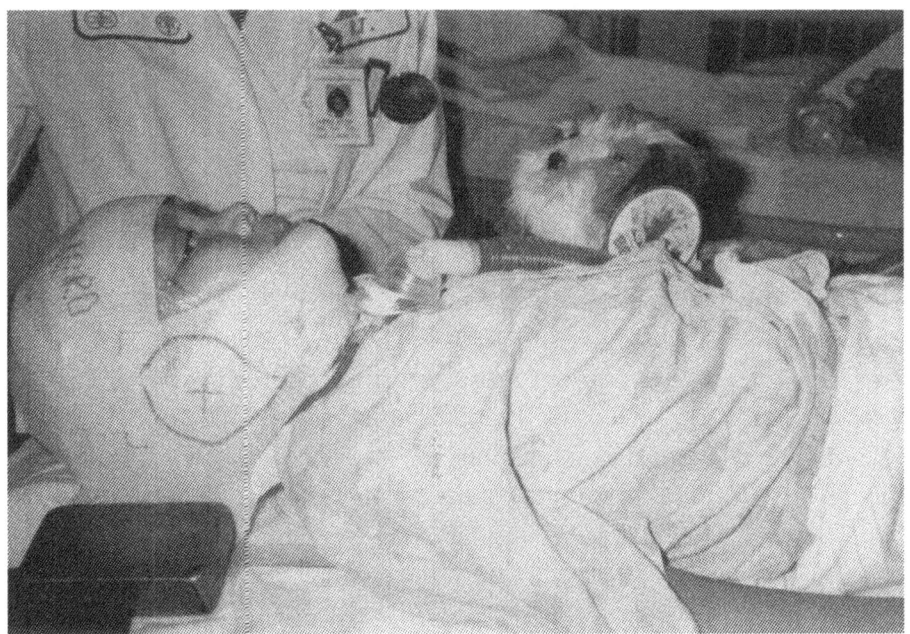

Andrei during radiation treatments

Chapter 7

Family and Test of Faith

Christmas of 1989 was approaching. I decorated the area surrounding Andrei's crib with Christmas decorations. It looked very festive and he was excited because he had accumulated many gifts around his miniature Christmas tree. We had the most amazing New Year's Eve, which eventually was our last one together; maybe Andrei sensed it. He always fell asleep by 11:00 p.m. but, on that particular night, he stayed up until 2:00 a.m. We watched the Dick Clark show and one of his favorite groups, "Expose," performed. The nurses brought me a cup of champagne and we happily brought in the New Year. As soon as the clock hit midnight, I grabbed Andrei and we embraced. My lovely supportive mother was also staying the night with me, which she tended to do often during the months we were at the hospital. She has always been there for me.

Let me elaborate about this incredible and amazing woman whom I am so fortunate and blessed to have as my mother. She's a strong woman who adores her grandson and daughter. She'd suffered enormously, having lost two of her own sons only eight months apart before Andrei's diagnosis. She knew what I was feeling and she wanted to be brave and strong for us. Although my mother was limited in assisting Andrei and me, due to her blindness, just her presence was good enough. I rarely discussed how awful I felt because I knew she was in pain and did not want to aggravate it.

Andrei adored my mother; I believe he loved her even more than me. When she would wash clothes, he insisted on carrying the basketload to her room, when she would walk down the porch steps he would hold her hand and guide her. Andrei called her "Nana" and "Mama" (I was "Mommy"). I worked nights so I would bathe him, put on his pajamas and leave the bottles prepared; my mother would stay with him until he fell asleep and, in the morning, he always called out for her.

Although Mother is blind, she washes dishes, clothes and even cooks. Mother also dyes her own hair, coordinates her clothes, applies her make up and even exercises on the treadmill because, after all, she does have her vanity. I believe the most fascinating thing about her is her personality; she has the enthusiasm and courage to live out her life regardless of her condition. She carries herself with the utmost energy and spirituality. I recognize that a great deal of my strength and courage comes from my role model, my mother.

My grandmother, Ernestina, Andrei's great-grandmother, who was very elderly, would make the effort three times a week to visit us; her health started to deteriorate more with Andrei's illness. She loved him deeply and it would tear her apart seeing him in this crib unable to run around. She would not hide it, either, she would utter, "This is killing me, I can't handle seeing him like this, I can't bear it."

Grandmother was also very spiritual, constantly praying and having much faith in a miracle. The positive energy was spread to her daughter (my mother) to keep up the faith and hope; she also emphasized to me to be strong.

My father, Francisco, visited on a daily basis. He'd come in the morning and leave in the afternoon before traffic hit, occasionally taking my mother back with him so she could shower and rest. However, Mom usually insisted on staying nightly with me, also sleeping in a chair. Andrei called my father by the name of "Tata" and had a special gesture for his Tata. When my dad would grab his lips, Andrei puckered them. Dad kept a positive attitude, never allowing us to see the real pain he was feeling. He had already lost his two sons and seeing his grandson fighting for his life was painful.

My sister, Linda, brought my clothes to me; I would shower at the hospital in a room they provided for me. My sister and my brother Frank, were very special to Andrei. They both had baptized him in a Catholic ceremony. They were very supportive, loving, caring and never let us down. I could always count on them both and it was a great satisfaction and comfort to know that. Frank and Linda would make Andrei smile often, play and goof off with him. They bought him many gifts and filled his room with toys. My nephew, Augustine, the son of my eldest brother Augustine was also a very significant person in Andrei's life. They loved each other and I know Andrei felt a tender, special love for Augustine.

The morning of New Year's Day, Sebastian made another appearance at the hospital, carrying an enormous bag full of Christmas gifts for Andrei. He asked me to step outside to talk to him; he then sat me on his lap and had tears in his eyes. He told me that he wanted to get his act together and be around more often. I cried with him and told him he had to make an effort because I did not have patience with his behavior. He was not consistent and it was going to hurt Andrei. I told him I thought he was not a bad person, but too easily influenced by his parents. If he did not break away, he was going to regret it and resent them in the long run.

As Andrei's third birthday approached, I went across the street to the mall to purchase a gift. I bought him a Snoopy personalized birthday greeting card and a large stuffed animal, but when I approached the cashier, I began to cry.

I told the salesgirl, "Today, my baby turns three years of age and he has had to endure so much, he's hospitalized across the street and I do not know if this is going to be his last birthday with me."

The salesgirl began to cry with me. I needed to say something to a stranger in order to vent my emotions because I would never allow my family to see me suffering. I was always trying so hard to maintain a positive attitude and faith.

That day, I had a small birthday party for him in the playroom; there were pizzas and a cake and balloons. Some children from the ward attended as well as nurses and doctors, my family was there and my good friend, Muriel, helped. I videotaped the party and Andrei seemed happy but quiet.

Although I had a lot of faith, I honestly can say there were days when I questioned my faith. I could not comprehend how God could allow this to happen to innocent children. Why did children have to endure so much pain and suffering?

Some days I was rebellious and very angry with God to the extent I would not pray or ask Him for anything because I felt he was not listening to me. What also would upset me was seeing other children being discharged from the hospital and instead of feeling contentment for them and their parents, I was upset and jealous. Because all I could see was that maybe we were never going to leave or maybe Andrei was never going to get better.

My emotions were confusing. I went through this stage for a couple of weeks and, fortunately, snapped out of it. I needed to remain positive, and particularly, I needed to have faith in God that He was getting us through these difficult times. But I am human and these feelings are all part of human emotions.

At times, I tried playing for Andrei videotapes of himself and it would upset him, he would ask me to turn them off. I realized that it was disturbing for him not to be able to walk again, and it was ripping me apart that I could not do anything about it. My baby was hurting!

A little girl about three years old was also hospitalized with a brain tumor. She was in the bed next to Andrei, the following morning she was going to have surgery and a biopsy. She came out of surgery fine, only a portion of her hair was shaved off and the tumor was benign; within a few days she was released to go home, a very healthy girl. Once again, I was jealous, I wanted that child to be Andrei. I questioned everything and could not comprehend why he had to be the one with the malignant brain tumor, "Why my child?" I asked God and the world in general.

During the following days, the doctors began telling me of the wonderful possibility of Andrei coming home. It was a miracle, not even the doctors believed he would live this long and be able to go home. Finally, it seemed my prayers were being answered.

Although Andrei's diagnosis remained the same, the doctors were going to allow him to be nursed in the surroundings of his own home. He no longer required a respirator to breathe, one of the primary reasons for keeping him hospitalized. However, the oxygen was needed and that could be provided in the home.

The condition Dr. Hensley asked of me was that she wanted me to attend psychotherapy in order to deal with Andrei's illness. She was concerned with my attitude, dependency and strong attachment to Andrei. I was in denial of his terminal illness and was a one hundred percent dedicated mother, unlike other parents who would leave their child and come back in the morning. I couldn't see myself doing this; I never wanted to leave my son's side or have him sense not seeing me around for a long period of time.

Andrei would receive respiratory treatments and, several times during the day, they would suction his trachea after dripping a few drops of saline water. The suctioning consisted of sterile gloves and a thin plastic tube that was placed down into the trachea hole to draw up the phlegm. I always looked away because it was too difficult for me to watch.

One day, one of the nurses advised me to look on so that I could learn and begin to do the suctioning. I gave the nurse a nasty look and said, "I could never have the strength and courage to do this to my son and I will never learn."

Amazingly enough, a few weeks later, I was standing next to Andrei's crib when the respiratory therapist walked in. Out of the blue, I said to him, "Teach me, I want to learn."

He was stunned and quickly went to it before I changed my mind. I learned rapidly and from that day forward, when I was around, I was the only one Andrei permitted to suction him.

Andrei would receive arburteral treatments; these were respiratory treatments consisting of placing medicated drops into his trachea to clear the lungs. The respiratory therapists were very warm towards Andrei and, when they came into the room to administer the treatment, they would say, "Hi Andrei, it's time for your treatment, this is not going to hurt. It's going to help you breathe, OK."

On one occasion, a male therapist came in and totally ignored Andrei beginning the treatment as though he was unaware or cognizant. I was watching Andrei and realized he did not like the therapist's attitude and disliked being ignored. When the therapist finished the treatment, Andrei looked at him and pouted, his mouth made a verbal noise that sounded like buzzing, as if to speak. He was angry and was giving a signal as to say, "Hey, I am sick, but human."

Patients are sometimes treated just as that and we must remember they are human and deserve to be treated with kindness and respect.

I named his G-Tube 'Joey,' so that Andrei could relate to this foreign tube hanging out from his stomach as his friend. He would hold the tube and we would feed him his regular feedings, which consisted of a certain milk with all its nutrients that had to be added as a powder. Andrei also began to develop seizures and the doctors had to administer medication; the pain specialist doctors also came in to observe Andrei. Since cancer is such a painful illness, the doctors believed Andrei needed Valium to relieve some of the anxiety they felt he was experiencing.

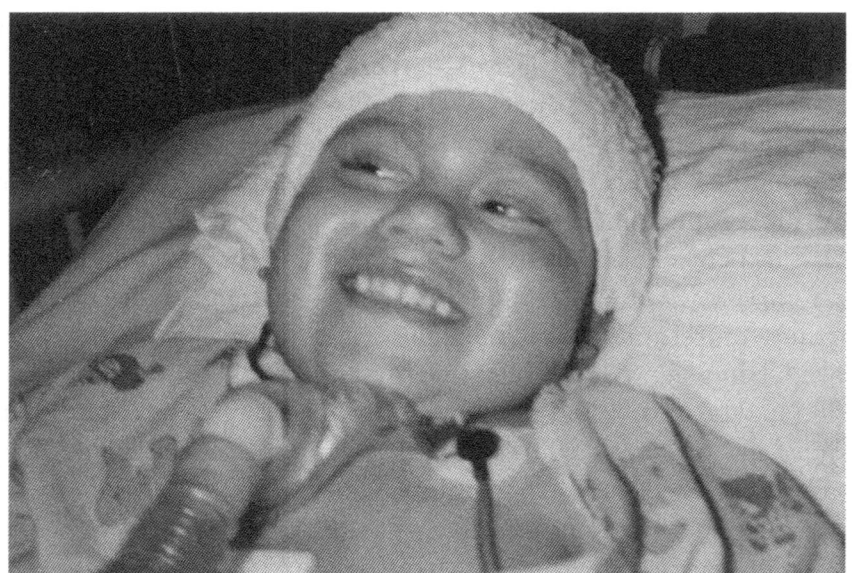

Andrei in the hospital

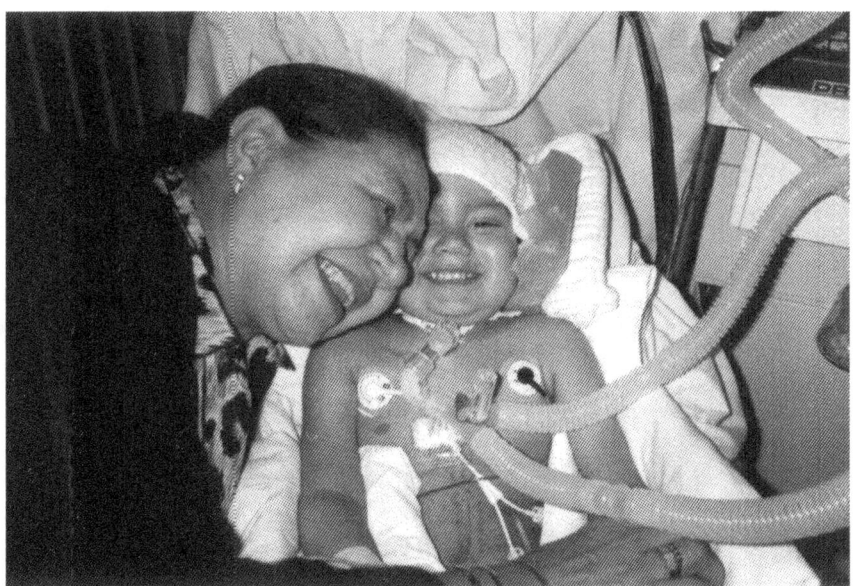

Andrei and Nana in the hospital

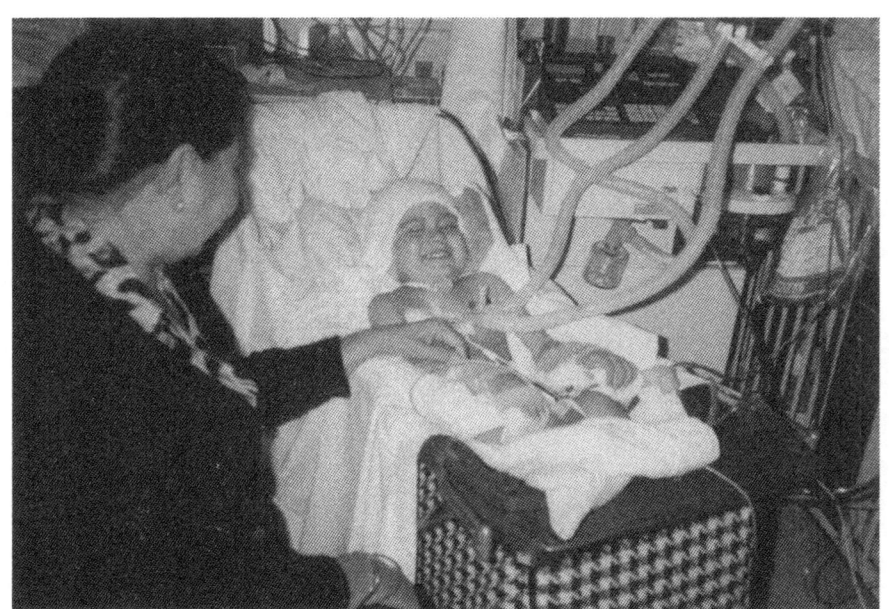

Andrei and Nana

Chapter 8
The Homecoming

The weeks passed and I began to prepare for Andrei's arrival home; a wondrous day that my family and I had been anticipating for a long time. I had to rearrange his bedroom to make room for the equipment (aprea monitors, pulse oximeter, IVAC pumps, Keogh feeding pumps, etc.). In addition, Andrei had already outgrown his crib and needed a bed. I began to leave the hospital for a few hours, leaving Andrei in the care of my mother, father and nurses. I constantly called the hospital to check up on him and assure him over the telephone that I would be there soon.

Andrei was going to need twenty-four- hour nursing care so we made arrangements with the insurance company, which hassled me with a lot of paperwork and faxed letters from the doctors. The insurance was only going to provide coverage for the first two weeks and then they were going to reduce it to twelve hours weekly, so I got assistance from the state. I also wrote to my congressman who helped with letters to the insurance company. The day crew was going to be provided by the state and the night crew was going to be the nurses of the Pediatric Intensive Care Unit at Cedars. I was content to know those nurses were going to work with us at home. Andrei knew them and this would help in the transition.

I hired a psychologist as instructed and the house was ready for Andrei. Angela, the nurse who owned the home care nursing agency, came up to me and told me she was going to be the nurse to assist me with Andrei on our way home. A nurse by the name of Paulina was close by, who had never been assigned to look after Andrei, when he pointed to her and said he wanted her to be the one. Paulina was one of the nurses who was going to sign up for the home care work; however, Andrei had never been treated by her but something about her drew Andrei to her. She was a kind African-American woman, she had a beautiful soft voice and later played a significant, loving role in Andrei's life; he grew to absolutely adore her.

During our five months spent in the hospital, I saw children come and go and some tragically die. I made new friends with many mothers whose children got well and others who died. I also realized many mothers were in the same situation I was in, without the support of the fathers of their children, and these women were married. There were a few couples who were blessed and together fortunate to have each other's love and support, which brought them together, closer and stronger.

The blissful day arrived and we were tense, anxious and excited. Andrei was very silent as though he was scared to leave the hospital. It was our sanctuary and the only surroundings we had become accustomed to since his surgery and paralysis. Andrei was finally weaned off the respirator and onto oxygen so we could have him on portable and stationary oxygen. The nurses and doctors came in to say their good byes. We packed our belongings and were on our way to a new beginning. God was granting us a second chance, and I was going to make the most of my time with Andrei with my family's support and love.

Our loved ones greeted us at home, and Andrei was placed in his bed and hooked up to the necessary equipment. I wanted him to be happy because he was away from the hospital and in his home, but he was not happy. He was crying and scared, he did not want to be home. His room now had more toys and photos to make him feel comfortable. My family and I tried very hard to help him adjust; it took about three days, then he was fine.

The hospital was our home away from home and the new friends we made were persons who were caring and loving towards us. Sebastian came over in the evening and wanted to be at the house for Andrei's homecoming; he was nice enough to buy Andrei a television set, VCR and many cartoon videos for his room. I pleaded with Sebastian not to mess up again since this day was so important to us and he promised he wouldn't. Sebastian came around for the first weeks after Andrei's release from the hospital and then, once again, vanished.

It was emotionally overwhelming having Andrei home because we were so incredibly happy. In the mornings, I'd walk into his room and yell out, almost in an operative voice, "Andy Pandy," my new nickname for him. He would light up with an enormous smile. Andrei and I began to bond as never before; we were growing into a very serious, mature relationship as mother and child and we were going to have to have strength and energy to fight the cancer. Andrei fought hard every day and, as far as I was concerned, he deserved every joyful moment life had to offer.

One day, we rented the movie "My Left Foot," with Daniel Day Lewis and watched it together. It was incredible how attentive he was to the movie. I observed this, turned to him and said, "Andrei, see how he could not walk and now he can, so can you. Just have faith in God, you will walk again." Since the actor could not walk at the beginning of the movie and walked at the end, it was a positive message.

We made numerous visits back to the hospital when Andrei's white blood count would be very low due to the chemo. His life was always at risk since he could contract any life-threatening illness with his immune system so susceptible. I know people questioned my ethics when they saw Andrei and me on our "special trips." I would load my car with portable oxygen tanks and we would go to the beach just to hear and see the waves.

One day we were watching 'The Munsters' on television and Herman Munster was playing a guitar. It totally captivated Andrei's attention and he gestured to me that he wanted one. Within the next few days, I loaded Andrei into the car with his afternoon nurse, Mindy, who later turned out to be a very dear friend to me. We parked in the lot at Toys-R-Us and I turned to Andrei, saying in a not–so- confident voice, "You want to stay here and wait for Mommy, I am going to go buy the guitar I promised you,"

He shook his head and said, "Yes."

All of a sudden I thought things over, turned to Andrei, extremely confident, and said in a loud voice, "Come on, Andrei, go with Mommy and let's get your guitar, OK."

That's what it took to change his mind. I observed that, since I was unsure of myself he reacted to those vibes but, once I was certain, he picked up on that just like everything I had been doing since he was diagnosed with the cancer. Positive thinking and positive action made an enormous impact. I placed him in a shopping cart with his car seat and the oxygen tank hanging on the side. I looked at Mindy and we both took a deep breath and said, "Lets do it."

My ultimate concern was that I did not want people staring at Andrei or feeling pity for him; I did not want him to feel uncomfortable. I took the cart and we walked into the store. It was amazing how people were so tactful; they did not stare. One gentleman came up, pushed me aside and told me I should be thankful to God Andrei was not on a respirator, which would make things worse and I would not be able to even go out-doors. He admired me for my courage.

Everything Andrei pointed to and said he wanted, we threw into the basket. We passed the Batman automobile that was on display. I pointed to it and promised Andrei I would buy it for him if he learned to walk again with the physical therapist. We had a two hundred dollar spree but it was worth every penny seeing how the smile lit up Andrei's face.

On another day, I wanted to take Andrei to Santa Monica to see the statue of the Blessed Mother near the beach. I wanted to take Andrei for religious reasons. The nurse that the state provided for us called in sick and the other shift was not due at work until 11 p.m. I somehow got courageous and my mother and I took Andrei to see the statue and we prayed briefly. We also went through the drive-through at Andrei's favorite place, McDonalds, to buy a children's meal.

I now reflect and question if I had been acting irresponsibly, what if Andrei had had problems breathing? I am so glad I did not think about those things because we would have never made the best of times if we did not take chances. If I had thought everything out, we would have not been so adventurous. My self-interest to see my son happy, if only for a few hours, out weighed the glances and fears that lurked behind the stares of strangers. *How could that mother take the chance of bringing her sick child out of the confines of home or hospital.* You see: their fears were not my fears. I needed to have Andrei enjoy every moment of life. My mother was also encouraging and participated in our daring acts. We drove back home and the night shift nurse was expecting us; we had a tremendous and unforgettable evening.

When I would catch a cold I could not go into the room without a surgical mask, in order for Andrei not to get sick with his low immune system. I would stay away as much as he would allow me. I would say to him, "Just wait until mommy's no longer sick, I am going to walk in here and kiss you starting from your toes till your head", he would smile. Then, when I recovered, I would do precisely that; he would get a kick out of it and laugh and enjoy me grabbing and smothering him. Many times I would kiss him frequently, repeatedly confirming to him how much I loved him. I would always be thankful for having that precious moment and lived that to the fullest; not aware of knowing if tomorrow he would be around.

Eventually, Andrei learned to talk through his trachea, although his voice was soft but understood. This allowed us to have more communication with each other. Andrei learned to identify his colors in Spanish and English; he also learned to count in both languages. I frequently gazed into his eyes and say to him, "You are my life! You are my world Andrei."

He would look straight into my eyes and reply, "No, Mommy, you are mine!"

I would ask Andrei, "What is your name?" and he would strain his voice through the trachea to say proudly and loudly, "Andrei Momero," because he could not pronounce his last name well.

He was just a very funny child who knew how to make the best of his time with this whole situation. On several occasions I would turn to Andrei and say, "Tu eres mi baby", (You are my baby) and he would answer rapidly in Spanish, "No, Mommy, Yo soy hombre", (No Mommy, I am a man).

Incredibly, he was an adult in a little boy's body. He amazed me with his characteristics, his sense of maturity and handling his illness to the best of his capabilities.

I was forced to return to work after six months, since I did not want the insurance carrier to cancel me. Andrei had dual coverage (Sebastian's and mine) but the medical bills continued to rise. My boss, Mr. Rogelio Dante, was a father himself and very compassionate towards my situation. During my absence from work, he continued paying my salary in order for my financial problems not to get any worse. I was excluded from working my two days off unlike the rest of the personnel who were obligated, due to lack of personnel on the airport evening shift.

Andrei was admitted into the hospital quite frequently because his immune system (white blood cell count) was low, causing caused numerous infections. The antibiotics would take about a week to function in his body. He'd have high fevers and there was always the chance that the medicine would not cure him. The procedures were the same, long and tedious.

Our attitude remained optimistic, although many days our energy level was low and we were exhausted from staying up all night. Fortunately, since Andrei had already outgrown the crib, he was now provided with a single bed which made things a bit more comfortable for us. I no longer had to sleep in a chair but I was able to sleep beside him in the hospital in his bed. The nurse, who would check his pulse and change the I.V., antibiotics, or oxygen, always awakened us.

During this time, the assistant manager at the airport, Mr. Victor Arriaga and Consuelo, a co-worker, were not very supportive and were quite uncivil to me. Mr. Arriaga was a large man, over six feet tall with a very rugged face, so he was quite intimidating to me. He made me nervous and uncomfortable because at work he would talk behind my back to the other employees, saying he could not count on me to show up at work most of the time and treating me in a frivolous manner. Consuelo backed him up one hundred percent and on one occasion, she took me towards the back of the office to state her opinion, which was that she believed it to be unfair that I was not working as much.

I replied, that I would change into her shoes anytime so that I would not be going through my situation. I informed her our employer did not have a problem with this, why should she? She saw my composure and realized I was not going to argue or battle it out with her. When she said, "Oh, but Sebastian left you," she really hit below the belt, but I did not let her know that. I calmly told her I never wanted to ever speak to her again unless it was work-related. I left for the bathroom and just burst out crying. My other co-workers caught up with me, told me to compose myself and not to let her know she got to me.

The only reason I did not sue for harassment was because I owed my boss, Mr. Dante, who was so compassionate. He would tell me, "I am your boss. As long as I am OK with everything, that is what matters."

I was not going to do something that would eventually reflect back on Mr. Dante and affect him in some way. He and his wife were caring and compassionate people, they were aware this was the best way they could assist me in my dilemma.

Since I have changed and grown so much, on looking back at this time, I feel I should have dealt with it differently. Getting out of the house and working was my only means of some normality in my life, it kept my mind preoccupied. I should have stressed how impossible it was for me to work under these conditions and maybe pleaded with them to make it easier on me, but my pride would not allow it. I felt I could not expect anything honorable from these people, but I could be wrong.

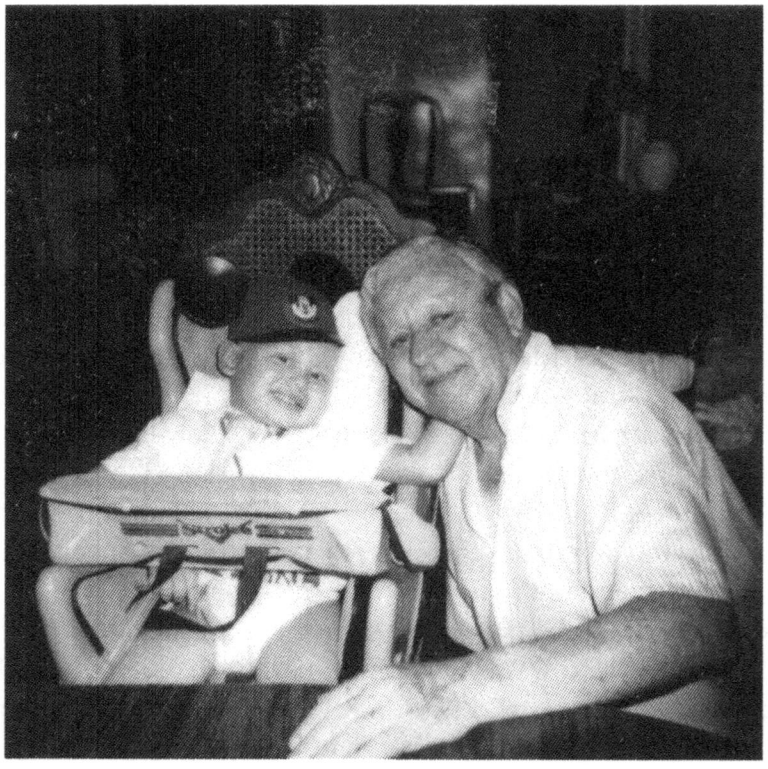

Andrei and Tata at home

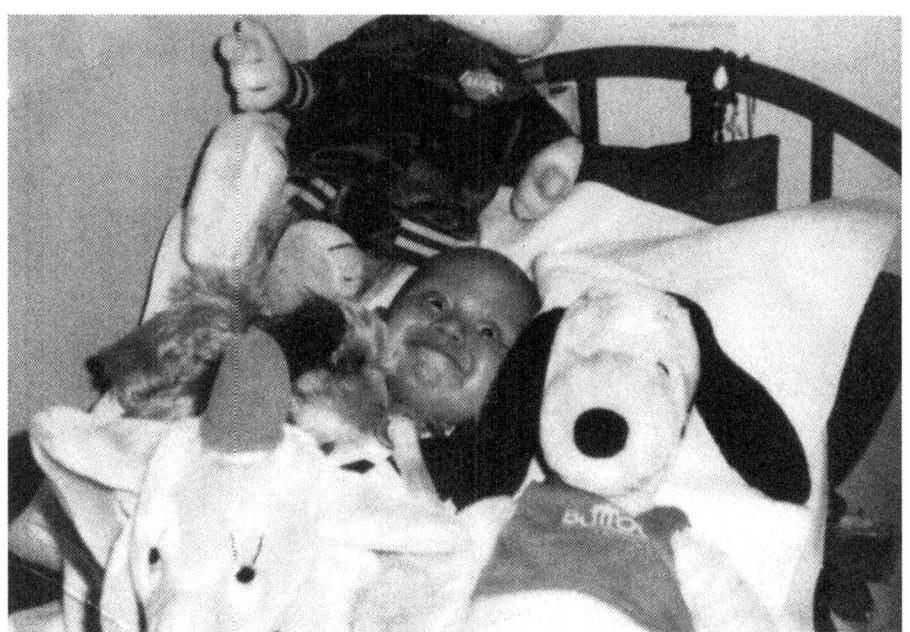

Andrei happy with his friends Snoopy, Benji , Dumbo and Bugs Bunny

Chapter 9

Andrei and His Nurses

There were various experiences with nursing staff. Since Andrei was receiving most of his nutrients via the gastrostomy tube (G-Tube), all of his medication was crushed and fed through the tube. One pill had a coating, making it impossible to be crushed. The pill needed to be substituted with a tablet that did not have the coating so it could dissolve.

During one of Andrei's stays at the hospital, I had my father go to the pharmacy to have Andrei's medication refilled and noted that the pill had to be substituted. Obviously, they called Dr. Hensley to authorize the change but the one in charge was the doctor's nurse. The nurse had apparently received the call from the pharmacy and felt inadequate and not knowledgeable. She came into Andrei's room as we were getting ready to head for home after recovery from another infection. She began yelling at me, asking me what I thought I was doing by changing the pill. I explained to her I needed something that could dissolve because Andrei's G-Tube had to be replaced twice because the pill was clogging up the tube due to the coating. She was so angry, which was due to her inadequacy, she just turned around and walked away.

Later that afternoon, Dr. Hensley walked in to discharge Andrei and I told her of the incident. She excused the nurse by saying the woman was stressed out. I replied angrily, "What do you think all these parents feel;

we are all stressed out and do not need someone to add to it. Her stress does not compare to ours and I never want her to talk to me that way again." The doctor said that she would talk to her.

Now I believe I should have made her come to apologize to me or refused to see her. Our insurance pays thousands of dollars to these hospitals and doctors so we have the right to obtain the proper, most professional and humane care possible. The social worker of the hospital for Andrei's ward was Georgina, a very nice, kind and caring person. I talked this over with her and said how upset I was. Another mother overheard and sided with me, saying she also felt this particular nurse, Dr. Hensley's assistant was arrogant and rude. Georgina was going to make Dr. Hensley aware of the complaints. I never found out what happened.

*　　　　　　*　　　　　　*

As the months passed by, Andrei was becoming more alert and also demanding, particularly of my time. He always wanted me beside him. One day he was home in his room with my mother and Cathy, another one of his favorite nurses, who would prepare peanut butter and jelly sandwiches and let Andrei have picnics with the neighbors' grandchildren. One of them Andrei considered his best friend, Louie. Andrei did not frighten them, especially with all his tubes as some children could become.

Cathy was also the nurse who took the initiative to have Andrei seated at the dining room table when it was my parents' wedding anniversary. Andrei at that time had just been released from the hospital and I was afraid to take him away from the confines of the bedroom. She said it would be okay so we got his car seat and sat him in it with his portable oxygen next to him. Andrei had the biggest smile on his face; he was so happy he could join us at the table and be a part of the celebration.

One day we were outside in his customized stroller and portable oxygen so that he can receive fresh air. I needed to go down the street to the drugstore to purchase some items. I asked Cathy to go with me and bring Andrei. When we arrived at the store, there was a car that operated by quarters. I sat in it first and then Cathy put Andrei on my lap and we put in the money. It was a blast. We kept putting money in the slot and laughing due to the excitement of it all. These are the precious moments I treasure, the goofiness and silliness we had together.

Cathy was wonderful with him but, one day, I guess he was frustrated when she was giving him a treatment and told her out loud, "Get out,"

He had already learned to talk better through his trachea.

I overheard and told him to apologize to Cathy, who did not deserve to be spoken to like that because she loved him very much. My stubborn child turned to me and said, "No", and pouted.

I was stunned with his rebellious side since he did not like to be away from me very long. He had become very possessive and demanding of my time. A child needs his or her mother around constantly for love, support and as a protective shield from the fears they have with unexpected changes taking place in their lives.

Nevertheless, I believed Andrei needed to have some normality of discipline in his life. My mentality was I believed he was going to get well and he was going to be so spoiled with all the attention he had been receiving, he later would not want to mind anyone. I told him, "Mommy is going to be in the living room watching TV and when you are ready to say you're sorry to Cathy, I will come back in the room to be with you."

I knew this would get to him because he could not stand being away from me. Twenty minutes passed. I checked in on him and told him I missed him but needed to know if he was ready to apologize and he said "No."

One hour went by and he finally gave in, it was so cute, he put his eyes down as though very embarrassed and said, "I am sorry." I kissed him and told him I was very proud of him for apologizing to Cathy.

Chapter 10

Beautiful Character

One of Andrei's other selected nurses was Estela, she was also very caring and loving towards him. One day I was working, and my mother said she was in the room with Andrei and Estela. I would not arrive home from work until almost 3:00 a.m. but Andrei would not go to sleep because he was waiting up for me. My mother was concerned and stayed with him until he could fall asleep but she was falling asleep herself. Three seconds after she did, Andrei pulled her head towards him and gave her a kiss on the forehead. He displayed tenderness and was very affectionate.

Andrei also disliked physical therapy. We tried to encourage him but he would act like he was asleep when the physical therapist would walk in. It was so funny. I thought one day he was actually asleep. Later when I said, "Andrei, they're gone you can wake up now," he did. I promised him to buy him his Batmobile at Toys-R-Us if he continued with the therapy, wanting to motivate him I told him we would walk in together to buy the car. It worked and he cooperated with the therapy.

The therapy helped. One day we sat him in my mom's lap and he began to swing back and forth. When he saw how excited we were, he kept doing it more and more. He also had movement only in his right arm, making it possible for him to make drawings for me, all the while favoring his left arm. He took much care of his arm, constantly embracing it with a tight grip for hours.

When I would do the chores around the house, my dad sat next to him and they listened to Frank Sinatra music on Andrei's Mickey Mouse cassette player. The amusing thing about it was that Andrei would say it was his Tata singing and nobody could talk him out of it. Since his right hand was the only one that was not paralyzed, he would change the cassette to the other side and push the play button; one of his favorite songs was "Chicago." Cecile and Paulina, the nurses with the charisma and voices to sing songs, would encourage him to sing with them. The environment that always surrounded him was energetic and charismatic. I can honestly say that, under the circumstances, we were happy.

One day the nurses attempted to discuss Andrei's passing away, but I would not hear of it. They tried through my sister, but I told Linda I would not give up on Andrei and did not want anything of the sort to be mentioned in the household that he could die. I never discussed dying with Andrei, although I would tell him often he was going to get better and he would become very serious and nod "No" to me on many occasions. I had a sensation he was aware of what dying meant because he would be firm and it was as though *he* needed to prepare *me* for his absence. It's difficult to explain, it was an inner feeling I sensed within myself.

Andrei had a beautiful charisma about himself, he was an adult in a child's body. He was strong and courageous, and his spirits were always high. Although he was paralyzed from the waist down after surgery, that didn't stop him from wanting to be in control of his own body and mind. Every morning he had to approve of his clothing. I would leave an outfit laid out for the nurse because I took him as an outpatient for chemotherapy; we needed to leave the house at about 7.00 a.m. I arrived home late and was not able to get to bed until 3.00 a.m. or sometimes 4.00 a.m. I made sure I left everything ready to leave early. When I 'd come into the room, Andrei would be wearing something different.

Then the nurse would tell me how he made her go through his clothes until he saw something he approved of.

At bedtime, the nurses would administer a medication by the name of chlorohydrate to help him sleep better. They would say, "It's time to give him the chlorohydrate" and he would pout and say, "No Mimi." That meant to him, "No sleep."

It was hysterical so we had spell the words out as a code so he did not know what we were up to. He was outsmarting us and was learning the medical terms at the same time. Andrei had outgrown his Pampers so there was no choice but to use small adult ones. He was upset and we could not get him to wear them; he thought they were big and ugly. If we tried putting them on, he would start crying. It took a lot of convincing and love to get him to wear them, since he could be very feisty and stubborn.

On our rides to the hospital, the nurse would sit in the back. We would put Andrei in the front and he was happy. He always wanted me to hold his hand, as I drove, most of the time that is exactly what I would do. When we'd see the big trucks, we'd indicate to them to honk, they were always so kind when they'd see Andrei and grant us that. The sad thing was when Andrei would see a car that looked like Sebastian's, he'd point and say "Mommy, Papa," in a sad voice. I'd say, "Yes, Andy, lets wave," and we would always wave at the cars. It was our routine every time we were on the freeway and the cars reminded him of his daddy.

After many incidents like these, I thought I would swallow my pride and call Sebastian to let him know Andrei has been thinking about him a lot. What made me make this decision was that I was also videotaping Andrei and I was asking him questions. We started on questions about what he wanted to do when he grew up and he said he want to play "b-ball," his abbreviation for basketball. He said his favorite team was the Lakers. I knew he was saying this because his daddy would watch basketball games on television with him.

I ask him what was he going to do with the money he earned playing b-ball. He said he was going to buy me a house and car. I'd ask him to speak into the video and say whom he loved, he went down the list and named everyone, then he said, "Mommy, and Papa?"

I always told Andrei during these months that Papa was working and could not come but Papa loved him very much. I told him to speak into the video to say how much he loved him; to my surprise Andrei responded upset and said firmly, "No."

He paused, then said, "He is at his house, he's not working, Papa is ugly, I want a pretty Papa."

It's like everything I had believed, he also thought. Andrei knew otherwise, even though we had been protecting him from the truth.

I called Sebastian at work. Five months had passed by and we had not spoken to each other so he was surprised to hear from me. I told him I wanted us to put aside our personal feelings and I needed him to come to visit Andrei, who was asking a lot about him and missed him tremendously. I said if it made him feel uncomfortable to come to my home because of the rift between my family and him, he could visit at the hospital. Since we were going on outpatient visits frequently, he would have access to visit us and not feel awkward. He thanked me for calling and said he would show up one day soon but he never did.

I never believed Sebastian to be so selfish and only focused on himself. My friends at work told me that he had requested a month "leave of absence" to cope with the situation. Apparently, he was breaking down at work when he would hear Andrei was back in the hospital fighting an infection. The boss granted him the leave, however Sebastian never made any attempt to visit or call Andrei.

I recall Sebastian telling me once during our courtship how he would throw himself in front of a passing car if it were going to strike me. I believed our love to be very special and that we would share a life together for many years and have many children since we discussed children often. I believed he would be a good father and husband. How mistaken one can be, I never imagined in a lifetime that Sebastian would abandon us!

On June 3, 1990, my grandmother, Ernestina, passed away from complications with her heart. I left work and stopped by the hospital to check in on her about 3:00 a.m. seeing she was all alone, I called my mother letting her know I would stay until someone could relieve me. I slept in the chair next to my grandmother and ask her to intercede for me when she was in Heaven so that Andrei could get cured.

My grandmother was on morphine so she never woke up; my mother and aunts came in the morning at 9:00 a.m. to stay with her. As soon as I arrived home they called me to say my grandmother had just died.

Grandmother Ernestina was an amazing woman who always wore scarves around her neck and bright red lipstick. She was very spiritual lady who lived life to the fullest and was always confident God would get us through every difficult time we experienced.

I went to Andrei to break the news and he looked at me as though he had already known, or as I believe now, that my grandmother came to say good bye to him. Andrei's great-grandmother adored him and it caused her pain to see him this way. I did not grieve my grandmother's death strongly, she was in her eighties and she had lived a long life. I was also preoccupied with Andrei's health, unsure if his life would be a long one. I was scared that my world was going to fall apart.

After her passing, I found a letter from my grandmother written to me. It was a beautiful letter in which she expressed her feelings about the pain she is aware I am experiencing and empathizes with what I have had to endure. The part I liked the best is where she gives me her blessing and tells me God is with me through all the pain to comfort me.

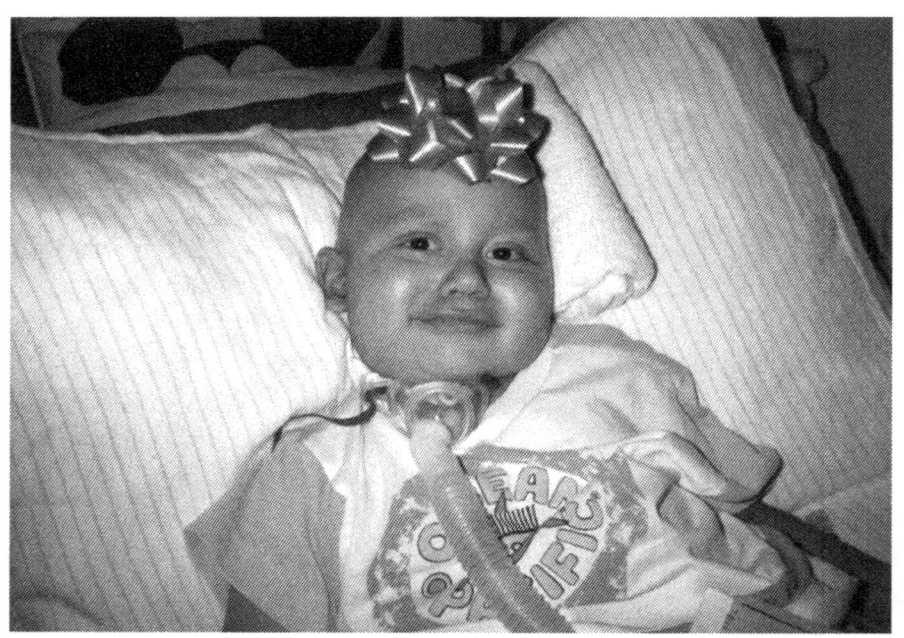

Andrei being goofy after opening a gift

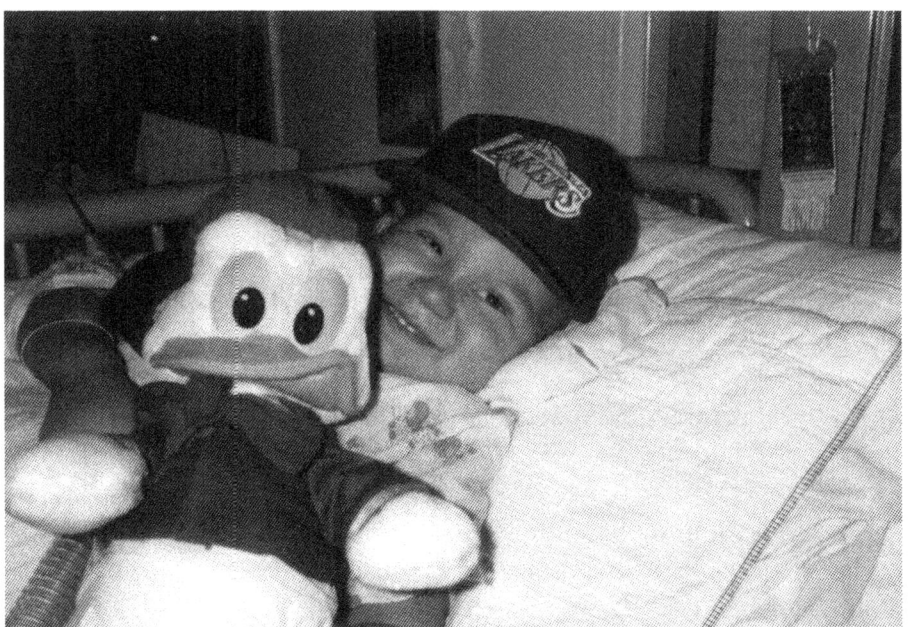

Andrei with his Donald Duck

Chapter 11

Time Drawing Near

On one visit, I ran into the doctor who had told me Andrei was not going to make it, and he was surprised we were still around. He actually told me it was a miracle and maybe Andrei's chances were favorable.

Dr. Hensley was also amazed with Andrei's improvements. The chemo was working and had shrunk the tumors that had spread to the lungs. They told me Andrei would be written up in a medical book because he was a patient who responded to those treatments. The tumor in his brain had maintained its size and had not grown.

The chemo was not causing Andrei to get sick. Dr. Hensley would come in now to see if his food intake might cause him nausea. Of course, we would order light foods for him like gelatin and soft food; once again, to her amazement, he never got sick. Andrei did lose his hair, his eyebrows and beautiful long eyelashes with the treatments. He always had such vanity when it came to his hair so he wore many baseball caps. One favorite was his Lakers cap; he also liked his Mickey Mouse T-shirts and socks.

Three months passed, and it was the month of September. One day, as we began to bathe him, I noticed he had a large bump on the back of his skull which we had not seen before. It did not feel right, so I called Dr. Graine, the neurosurgeon, and set up an appointment for Andrei.

We went the next day and I noticed as we waited in the waiting room that Andrei was nervous and scared. I assured him it would be okay and the doctor was only going to look at his new owie. He turned to me and said, "Tin is going to take away my owie,"

That was my eldest brother's nickname who had passed away when Andrei was eleven months old. I was stunned and knew my brother was with Andrei in these difficult moments. The doctor examined Andrei and hospitalized him for further tests; we were there about a week when I insisted they give me the new diagnosis.

While waiting for the new diagnosis at the hospital, we continued to be optimistic and prayed that it would not be something serious. Andrei was goofy and playful; his sense of humor was unique. One afternoon we were lying in the hospital bed watching television when the afternoon news came on discussing something about MRI studies. This word was familiar to Andrei because he had received many of them during the year. He started swinging his right arm and bopping his head side to side singing the lyrics "MRI, MRI".

I laughed and looked at him and said to him, "You are so crazy." We both began laughing together, then I grabbed him and smothered him with kisses.

It was fortunate we had so much fun together because the latest test results revealed the tumor was *larger*! And it was beginning to bulge out of his skull! Andrei did not have much time left. The doctors did not want to do surgery but they could raise his level of chemotherapy to higher doses. They allowed us to take him home until I decided what to do; the concern was that the higher doses of chemo were going to result in a lower immune system. I told my boss I was no longer coming back to work, that Andrei was critical.

My sister, Linda, began her research again and called many doctors for opinions. One in particular was a Dr. Eisner from New York. He was well known for avant-garde surgeries that pertained to these types of tumors, but we would have to fly Andrei to New York. We heard that

Mr. Donald Trump helped in these cases and allowed his airplane to be used, but the arrangements were difficult. I wanted second opinions so we called two other renowned physicians in pediatric neurosurgery, Dr. Blanchard and Dr. Palmer from UCLA. My family, Andrei, the nurse and I went to the appointment.

The doctors looked at and read his medical records; we took all the copies, even the x-rays. They wanted to know why I didn't bring Andrei to them in the beginning. I told them I tried but it was when they were in India and could not see us. They asked the nurse to leave with Andrei, and my nephew, Augustine, went with them to keep him company. I stayed with my parents and sister. The doctors looked directly at me and said, "Andrei has two weeks to live, approximately."

I started crying hysterically with my mother and could not believe this was really going to happen to us. The doctors said they could do the surgery but there were a lot of risks involved.

They wanted to go through Andrei's mouth and retrieve the tumor; the surgery could also cause meningitis. They allowed us to stay in a room so that we could cry and let it out before we would go out in the waiting room where Andrei was. We all put up a front and we did not allow Andrei to see us upset. We assured him of our love and put on a happy face all the way home.

All my friends, (Jennifer, Cassandra, Lourdes, Muriel and Christian), became very supportive. They visited to tell me that they were there for us for whatever we needed. Apparently, my boss told Sebastian that Andrei had only two weeks left and that he should make an effort to see him. I couldn't call Sebastian. I was so distraught and my focus was to make Andrei comfortable and happy the last days of his short life.

I myself was in denial and was definitely still expecting a miracle to happen.

Inez and Kevin Contreras were very dear friends who were introduced to me by Sebastian's parents, their friends of many years. They were very sweet and supportive. When they heard Andrei's prognosis, they asked if Inez' brother could visit with church members from their congregation. He belonged to a Christian church, played the guitar and sang Christian songs with four other gentlemen. They wanted to come and sing also pray over Andrei.

I immediately accepted and, to my amazement, the music really soothed Andrei, he absolutely enjoyed it. One day they left his room because he had fallen asleep and they did not want to disturb him; he woke up and demanded they come back into his room. He had begun to have strong headaches since the tumor was growing rapidly. He had already lost his voice since the vocal cords were now paralyzed due to the pressure of the tumor. But a miracle was occurring: When he heard the music he had no headache, God was carrying him in His arms and the angelic music eased his pain.

I continued to say to Andrei, "You are going to get better, you will be healed."

He would turn to me and firmly say, "No," again as though he still felt he was not going to get better. He also wanted me to accept the fact he may not make it and I needed to deal with it.

I remember even whispering in his ear, "Do not leave me, Andrei. You have to get better because Mommy cannot live without you."

I now feel so dreadful for saying this to him. It was not right to put him under that pressure but, as a selfish mother, I was not thinking clearly. If it was best for Andrei and his pain would no longer exist, I needed to learn to let go. We would all hold hands and pray together for Andrei's health and for my resignation. During those two weeks, we continued to be optimistic, happy and faithful a miracle might happen.

On one day my sister, Linda, rented a Batman costume so Andrei would believe he was really there visiting him. I put it on first and he was absolutely thrilled to see me. He kept reaching out to unveil me and prove it was his mommy since I kept telling him I was Batgirl.

We had fun. My sister, Augustine, my nephew and I acted very goofy to make the best of our time with him. For instance, we made a train chain and march around his room singing Disney songs. When Augustine came out with the costume, Andrei really believed it was Batman. His acting job was excellent and Andrei was fascinated while I videotaped everything. It was so silly but cute and that moment was one of the best for Andrei.

It was October 3, 1990, and the two weeks were drawing to a close.

A nurse had stepped out of the room to prepare Andrei's feeding. I was present as he stared hard at the ceiling, extremely attentive as if someone had spoken to him. I felt the presence of someone and got chills down my whole body. I looked at Andrei and asked him what was he looking at; he mouthed, "Mommy."

I replied, " But mommy is here."

He then grabbed his rosary which was hanging from his bed and mouthed, "Jesus Mommy."

He often would lay the rosary on his forehead to help his owie because I would tell him God was going to heal him. I knew then he was in the presence of the Blessed Mother. I told Andrei, "If she is here, blow her kisses," and he rapidly started throwing kisses up above him.

I called Sister Angela and that evening, with friends, we prayed the rosary. I questioned this and thought, "What does this mean, will he get well, or is the Blessed Mother here to prepare him for his next journey?"

On October 6, a Saturday morning, I looked at Andrei and he didn't look well. I turned to the nurse; "Do you think it's time?"

She replied, "No, it will be a few more days."

Somehow, call it mother's intuition, I knew time was running out. The tumor had practically bulged out of his skull. He couldn't be moved because it was so painful. Because of an inner feeling I had, I asked Andrei, "Can mommy hold you?"

He nodded his head "YES." I held him in my arms from 10:00 a.m. till 10:00 p.m. The entire day, I reassured him of my love while holding him tightly; he loved hearing about when he was a baby so I talked to him about it. The nurse from the night shift arrived. My mother convinced me to put Andrei back in his bed. I had not gone to the restroom nor eaten for the entire day. Thirty minutes later, Andrei had trouble breathing. We called for an ambulance.

Andrei was semi-conscious. The paramedic told me I could not ride in the ambulance with him, only his nurse. Thank God it was Paulina, the nurse he had requested to bring him home and now, ironically, was the nurse taking him back. I pleaded with the paramedic and told him, if Andrei woke, he would be devastated if he did not see me. He was compassionate and said it was against the law, but he was going to let me ride with him anyway.

As the siren sounded, he opened his eyes and asked, by mouthing the words, for Nana, Tata, Uncle Frank, Auntie Linda and JR, my nephew, Augustine. I assured him they were following us in another car and not to worry. I was trying very hard to hold back the tears, I felt my heart was ripping apart. Andrei held his Pink Panther stuffed animal during the whole time.

When we arrived at Cedars Sinai Hospital, Juliet, a Pediatric Intensive Care Unit nurse, told me Andrei was dying. She needed me to make the greatest ethical decision of my life, "Decide, now! Do you want him on life support machines."

I looked at my parents. Their eyes said, "This is your decision."

I left the room and went into the hall. I stood screaming and crying and hysterically pulling my hair! I could not believe this was really happening. I ran to the phone. I called Father Sean Cronin but his answering machine was on. This was my decision! No life support!

It was important to me that Andrei remained alert. I stuck to my decision and advised the nurses I wanted him alert until the last moment. If Andrei showed any indication of pain and suffering, I would allow the doctors to administer morphine for pain.

My mother told me Sebastian had to be called and I refused. She told me if I did not, I would regret it for the rest of my life. I then agreed and my brother, Frank, said he would make the call. He called him about

2:00 a.m. in the morning and told him Andrei was dying. Sebastian responded, "What could I do?"

Frank replied firmly, "Get over here and see your child."

But the hours went by and Sebastian did not show up. My co-workers came after work and began calling him but he let the answering machine pick up the calls. My friend, Rita, called and left an extensive message saying he had to come. She pleaded with him and told him he would have regrets if he did not do so.

At about 7:00 a.m. he appeared, distraught and scared. I will never forget the moment. He went to Andrei and said, "Your daddy is here."

Andrei looked away and never looked Sebastian's eyes again. The Christian men came to pray so Sebastian went and told them how he felt. When Sebastian left the room I looked at Andrei and said, "Yippee! Your daddy is here, aren't you happy?" and he nodded "Yes."

When Sebastian was not looking at him, Andrei would look for him throughout the room; he was extremely happy his daddy was there with him. I guess Andrei was trying to punish Sebastian for not being there for him because he would not budge. He just simply would not look into Sebastian's eyes when Sebastian placed his face into Andrei's, telling him he loved him.

Chapter 12

Andrei's Journey to Heaven
and My Final Goodbye

On October 7, 1990, Andrei was alert the entire day without visible pain and especially breathing on his own. In one of the drawers beside him, I found two gold colored electrodes (patches to hold the wiring for heart monitors) so I placed one on his shirt and another on mine. I whispered to him and said, "We both have a heart of gold" and kissed him. The doctor was even considering transferring him out of the Intensive Care Unit; he was improving and his breathing was better.

Father Sean Cronin appeared at 6:30 p.m. that evening. We prayed over Andrei and he was given the Sacrament of the Sick. During the prayers, Father Cronin referred to a section in the Bible that read, "the gates of Heaven will open to receive you," and then Andrei fell into a deep sleep. At 6:55 p.m., Father Cronin asked me to step outside the room for a moment. He told me Andrei was ready to go. Father said Andrei was holding on because of me and told me to let go. My friend, Muriel, immediately summoned me back into his hospital room because Andrei was calling for me. I walked in and he asked me to "suction" him.

As the nurse and I began the procedure, his breathing began to dwindle. I told the nurse to keep "bagging" him with the oxygen. The digital numbers on the side of the bed indicating his pulse rate were tapering off. The nurse turned to me with tears on her face and said, "Let him go Antoinette."

I was in shock. Her words meant nothing to me. I took the pump from her hands and began pumping, as the thoughts screamed in my head, "This cannot be happening."

Andrei, who had lost his voice due to paralyzed vocal cords, looked at me and miraculously was able to yell, "No more, Mommy." He was still holding his Pink Panther.

Shocked, I uttered the hardest words possible for any mother, "Go, Andrei, go to Heaven, your grandma and uncles are there waiting for you. Mommy will be okay."

The nurse quickly grabbed Andrei and put him in my arms, we sat in a chair as I wept and held him tightly until his last breath.

At 7.25 p.m. he was pronounced dead.

Sebastian came to us and knelt down beside us, asking me to forgive him, then he went to my parents and did the same. I just cried and cried and began muttering, "Andrei, I tried to give you the best life I could."

After a few minutes, the nurse told me I had to put Andrei on the bed because his body was going to stiffen. I reluctantly laid him on the bed when Dr. Hensley walked in. She was not on call, but she said she was paged. The nurses insisted she could have not been paged since she is never on call on weekends. It was very strange and, if she had not come, she would never have been able to say her good byes. Because Andrei was being taken to the morgue and would have not been there in the morning, maybe it was Andrei who made the pager go off.

Dr. Hensley mentioned how significant it would be to be able to perform an autopsy on the rare tumor, but she said she knew Andrei had already been through enough. She had tears in her eyes. I had discussed with the nurses at noontime that I did not know how I was going to react after Andrei's death. So, before I really lost my composure, I asked that, when Andrei died, that my brother Frank carry him downstairs to the morgue.

I had lived so many months in the Intensive Care Unit and experienced so many deaths; I saw parents leave and not be aware that their babies were being taken away on a small wheeled aluminum table, just lying on top. I did not want Andrei to be taken like that and the nurse assured me Andrei would not be treated in that manner. She said she and the whole unit considered Andrei to be very special, and he would be taken care of in a special way.

Dr. Hensley approached me gently and told me in a very kind voice that I was a wonderful mother and did everything possible for Andrei. She knew he loved me very much. She then left and all the nurses came in to say their good byes. We held hands, cried and prayed, my family and I later did the same. I was so distraught and numb; my life had fallen apart.

About 2:00 a.m. on October 8, the mortuary man came to take him away. Andrei was put into a black plastic bag with a zipper in the front and, before the man zipped him up, I grabbed him again and kissed him. I walked with the man towards the elevator and he told me I could no longer go with him. I cried and felt such a vast emptiness in my heart. Andrei and I were going to be separated for the first time from the time of his birth; he was no longer going home with me.

As we walked out, Sebastian looked so scared that I asked him if he wanted to go to our house. He quickly accepted. He later told me he was so grateful because he was so scared, in the last few days, he had slept with the lights on. Sebastian also thanked me for suing him for child support. He said if I hadn't done that, he probably would have not had the chance to get to know Andrei. It pushed him to request visitation rights.

I had about four days to prepare Andrei's funeral, and I wanted it to be very beautiful and special, graced with serenity and peace. I had been putting money away for Andrei in a savings account for college; ironically, it was the money for his funeral. I went to the bank to close the account. The bank teller made a comment, saying, "Are you sure you want to close this account."

I began crying and told her, "I wish I did not have to, this money was for my son's future and now I need to use it towards his funeral."

Her eyes became watery, she processed everything and handed me $2,500.00. It was an amount that would at least help me pay for some of the funeral that totaled about $5,000.00.

I ordered arrangements of flowers with the designs of Andrei's favorite cartoon characters, such as Snoopy, Mickey Mouse and Batman. I asked people to wear bright colors to his funeral because he was an 'Angel' and his departure was to Heaven. People who wanted to help were asked to send flowers for Andrei at his funeral. I purchased white doves and one hundred balloons to be released after the burial.

I bought Andrei a tie and jacket and went to the mortuary to drop off his clothing. I asked the woman there to please put the Batman under-wear on him, place his Mickey Mouse stuffed animal with him and I told her to put his Batman socks on him. When I said this she began to cry, then I cried with her. I ask if Andrei was there and she insisted he was at another mortuary and would be brought there at a later date. I believe he probably was there but that she was just afraid I might ask to see him.

My father and Sebastian went with me to pick out the coffin. I chose a white wooden one. I think I was in a daze the whole time. I made some pamphlets with Andrei's pictures on it and a poem inside. Sebastian told me his mom and dad were arriving from Costa Rica and asked how I felt, about them. I said they were welcome to attend the services. I was not going to hold any hard feelings against them because I wanted Andrei to have a peaceful farewell.

As I was sitting in my room writing the eulogy, Sebastian's sister, Yolanda, walked in. She approached me and said, "If you want me to leave, I will understand." I told her, "Andrei is gone, that is the only thing that matters."

We sat for awhile and talked about Andrei, she appeared a bit embarrassed or shameful since she was absent the whole time. Then she commented, "We never truly thought Andrei was going to die."

I believe that is a partial reason they never came around; they believed they would have plenty of time to reach out, never believing their actions would haunt them forever.

For the rosary I made pamphlets that read "Our Little Angel," with a picture of Andrei with a Winnie the Pooh stuffed animal, looking very assertive. Inside, it read:

"In memory of Andrei who was a beautiful child so full of the courage, strength, love, goofiness and stubbornness that gave him the will to live. Andrei, you have left this world physically, but your spirit will always be felt around us. You are now a beautiful blessed little angel up in Heaven with the presence of God our Father and the Blessed Mother. And the most glorious day for me to await is when my time comes and we will meet again and live eternal life together. I will love you forever. Mommy"

My Angel Andrei

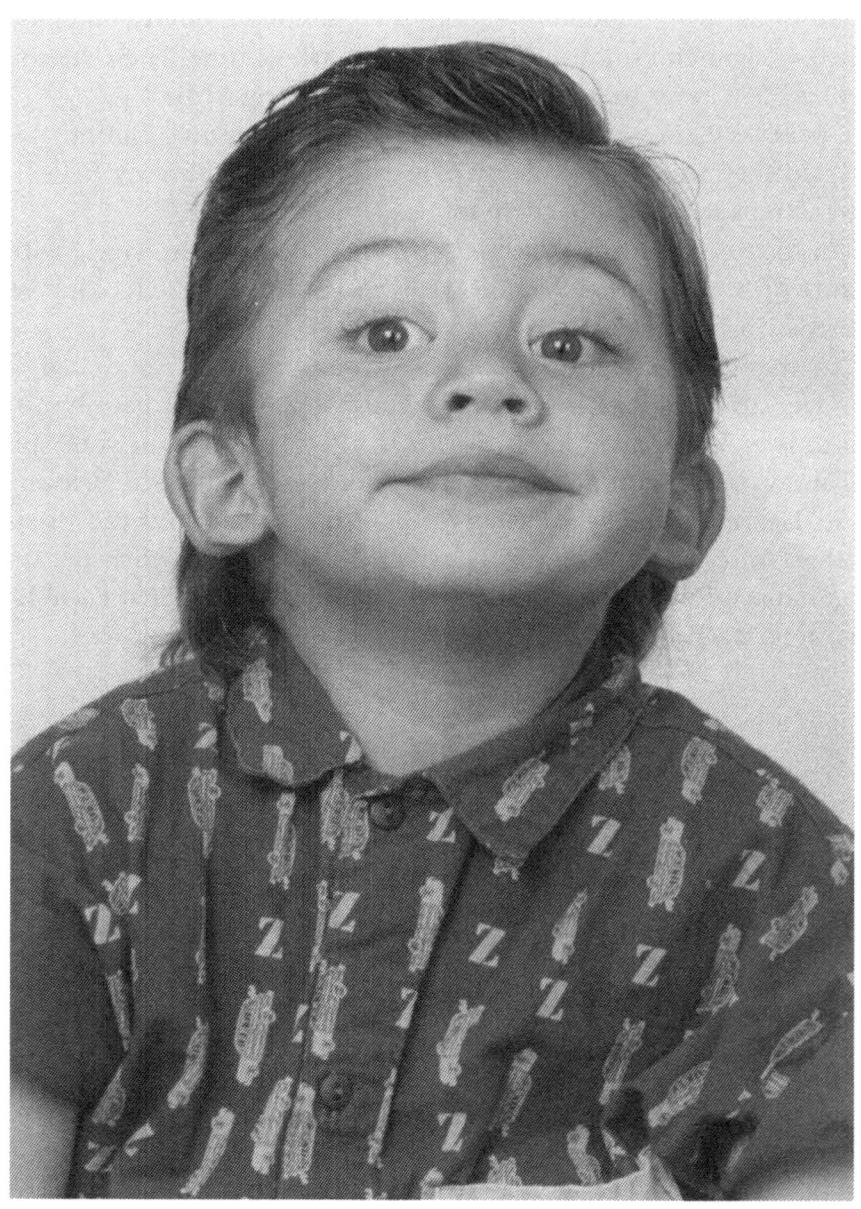

It also contained two other pictures on the back with his most frequent phrases in Spanish, "Yo, Batman" and "Mommy Te Quiero Mucho," translated to English, "I am Batman" and "Mommy, I Love You very much."

∗   ∗   ∗

Andrei's eulogy, written by me, and delivered by Sister Angela at the funeral mass, read:

CHERISHED MEMORIES OF ANDREI—OCTOBER 12, 1990. Andrei was born on January 4, 1987, on a Sunday; it was and is today still the most precious and blessed day of my life. As a baby, he was always so lovable and playful. As he began to grow, the little things he began to do brought so much joy and fulfillment into my life. When he became a toddler, there was so much pride within me because there was that independence and slight arrogance that made him so unique, he was developing into his little manhood personality. He had an adorable little strut when he walked which demonstrated a lot of self-confidence, how was I to know his little maturity was going to prepare him for the biggest experience and challenge of his little life. When Andrei was diagnosed with the brain tumor, I thought that my whole life was going to completely fall apart, especially after his major surgery. Andrei was beginning an enormous challenge for survival, he became a "fighter." Now I truly believe that he was not ready to go until he prepared me and touched the hearts of the persons who cared for him. Andrei hung in there for an entire year, to the amazement of family, friends, nurses and especially doctors. I remember a few days after his surgery he was still so critical, I would sleep next to him in a chair.

One day, about 3:00 a.m. I stood to check on him and then began to cry. He opened his eyes, looked directly into mine, threw me a kiss and smiled. I knew then that the message he was trying to get across was, "Mommy, don't cry, it will be OK." That is the day I began to have a very positive atti-tude and decided we were going to fight this cancer and win! Well, we did-n't win in the aspect that it didn't go away, but we gave it a hard time. We didn't let it take over our lives, after five months in the hospital we were able to go home; every three weeks Andrei received chemotherapy and never became sick from such strong medication.

At home, we truly made the most of everything. There were times we would go to the beach just so that he could see the waves; we had our adventurous trips to Toys-R-Us that pleased me so much when I'd see that big smile. Andrei was and will always be a very special child; everyone who came in contact with him felt a special bond. Even though Andrei became paralyzed from the waist down after surgery, that didn't stop him from wanting to be in control of his body and mind. Every morning he had to approve of his clothing and he could become very bossy towards the nurses and me. The joy and satisfaction that Andrei brought to everyone will always remain with us. About three weeks ago, Andrei was staring intently at the ceiling. I felt a sensation, asked him what he was looking at and he said "Mommy" and pointed to his rosary. When I asked him what color She had on, he said white; the beautiful Blessed Mother was in his presence as well as my late brother, Augustine, whom Andrei began to mention.

I'd like to give my thanks to my family for their strength and support, which played a big role in Andrei's life. Even though they were suffering, they never let him feel it. They were positive and showed him so much faith, love and courage. My special thanks to all the loving nurses who brought out the best in him; their love and dedication developed a special friendship with my family and I that will continue forever. Thanks also to all my caring friends who were there for me when I felt that coping with all of this was too overwhelming. Your dedication to me will always remain with me. My special thanks to my boss, Mr. Rogelio Dante, for all the con-sideration, only God can repay you for all your kindness. Thanks also to my co-workers for your loving support. A special thanks to Sister Angela and Father Sean Cronin. God Bless You All!

And now ,thanks to my beautiful loving son for giving me the honor to become his mother. Andrei, you are now a "little angel," who will be watching over me. When God calls upon me, we will meet again and live eternal life together. Andrei, was born on a Sunday and died on a Sunday, which is the Lord's day. Andrei you have taught a lot of us about life and courage, your spirit will always remain with us. I will always have you in my heart and no one will ever replace you, 'Andy Pandy.' God Bless, until we meet again! I love you forever, MOMMY.

The day came and the rosary was held. Father Cronin did a beautiful ceremony and gave Andrei a wooden star he had brought back from his trip to Bethlehem, indicating throughout the sermon Andrei was a star up in Heaven. People came up to us after the sermon to offer their condolences. When I looked up, I noticed a girl, one of Sebastian's friends, whom he had dated, and disliked me as much as I disliked her, coming towards him to shake his hand.

After the rosary, I had my last private time with Andrei. I went to the open coffin and cried as I stared at him and could not believe this was real. I bent down towards his face and said, "Oh, Andrei! Before when your dad did anything to hurt me it wouldn't hurt as much because I had you and now what do I do?"

I felt I had lost too much, my beautiful son who completed me and the man I had loved so much.

Some family and friends came to the house for coffee and snacks; I went to Andrei's room to cry and some friends stayed with me. My sister, Linda, popped in the videocassette of Augustine and me in the Batman costume, everyone was enjoying it. I got up to go to the restroom, as I passed by the hall I glanced to the dining room and to my astonishment, the girl was there. In my house!

I did not do anything even though my friend Muriel wanted to kick her out. I calmed down and realized she was not worth it, I would not lower myself to her level. My neighbor later told me that, as she was approaching the house, she saw them embracing. I was appalled to see she had no respect for my grief and pain, she had no business in my home. Sebastian also had no respect for the mother of his child because he was aware of my feelings and knew of my dislike for her.

The following morning the funeral mass was held at St. Peter & St. Paul church where both Andrei and me were baptized as babies. I had read the eulogy to my mother, translating into Spanish when Sebastian's mother and sister came over to the house. When Mrs. Carrillo heard what I was reading she began to cry, came over to me and said, "I am sorry for doing what I have done to you." These were the only words of compassion I had ever heard from this woman. I turned to her and said, "Mrs. Carrillo, the only thing I did was love your son too much and try to be a family." I was pleased she felt remorse and believed she meant it.

His sister, Yolanda, told me they always wanted to come to see Andrei and never believed he would eventually die, but that they thought I would not allow them to visit. I turned to them and said firmly, "But you never even made an attempt, you can never say you tried and I did not allow you to see him. I would have never turned you away from the doorstep, Andrei was your nephew and your grandson."

They felt sad and lost for words. The school choir sang at the mass, it sounded so beautiful and the Christians played their music at the burial site. I was told there were no dry eyes in the church after Sister Angela read the eulogy. Many people attended and Andrei was finally laid to rest.

It was now over and, soon after, the calls diminished. People believed I wanted to be alone but, in reality, I wanted to be accompanied by friends. Sebastian insisted on paying for the funeral but I declined because I did not want him to feel this was enough to clear his conscience.

A week after the funeral, Sister Angela told me a special mass was going to be held in memory of Andrei. The first-graders had been praying for him during his illness and were deeply saddened; they wanted to do this for me. Mrs. Carrillo attended the mass with me. At the school auditorium, the children held up an eight by ten photo of Andrei and sang beautiful songs.

We went to my home and I decided to take this opportunity to share my feelings with Mrs. Carrillo. I told her I was in deep pain, distraught on how I would now live my life without Andrei. She listened attentively. I felt I had to take advantage of this opportunity because this would possibly be the only appropriate conversation we might have.

I played the videocassette of my interview with Andrei in which he expresses the resentment he carried for his papa; she was speechless. Maybe it was cruel, but I needed her to know how affected Andrei was without his father in his life and she was to be also responsible for that.

Afterwards, I firmly told her that, after living through this ordeal and enormous loss, Sebastian had to learn a lesson. I expressed how unfortunate it was that he had to learn this way but I said I did not want Andrei's death to be in vain. Sebastian was going to be a better man, a better husband and father to another person and Andrei and I had to suffer the consequences for another woman and child to benefit.

Amazingly, she turned to me and said, " Antoinette, you never know, life creates many changes and that woman may just be you."

At times, I experienced desperate feelings, such as wanting to reconcile with Sebastian. I honestly felt if I would get back together with him and have another baby, it would have some similarity to Andrei and I would have my baby back. I knew nobody could replace him but I was desperate.

That evening, I wrote an entry in the journal that I had been writing in since Andrei's birth. It was my sad and tearful final good bye to my beautiful son.

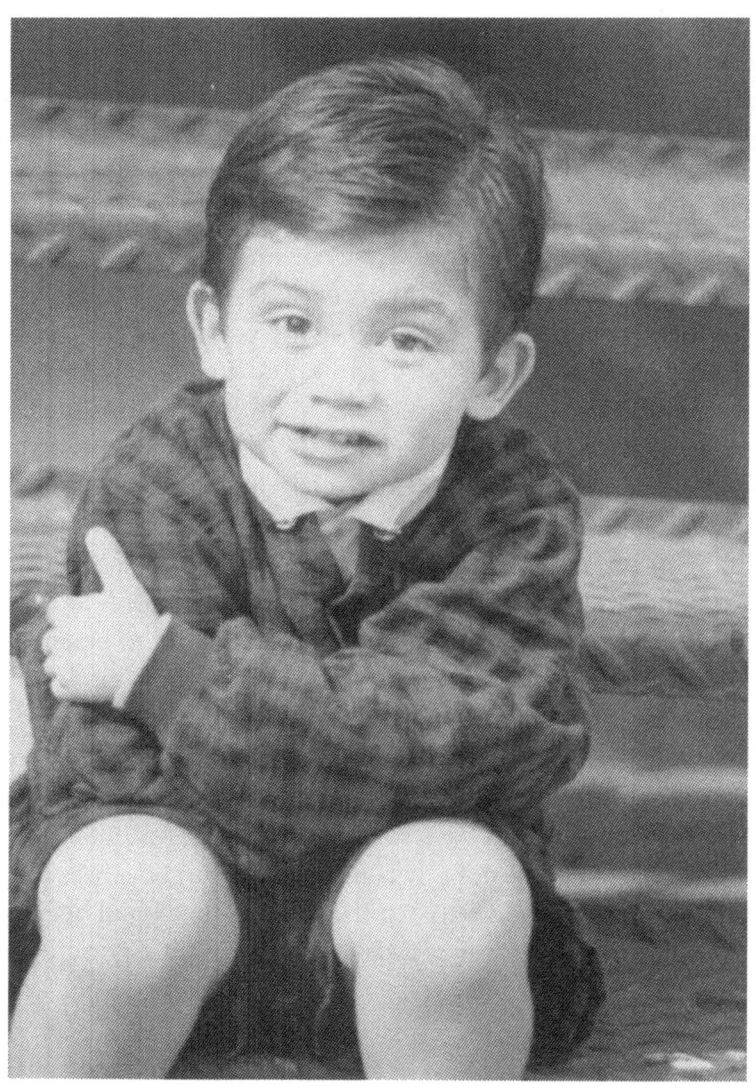

Andrei two and a half years old

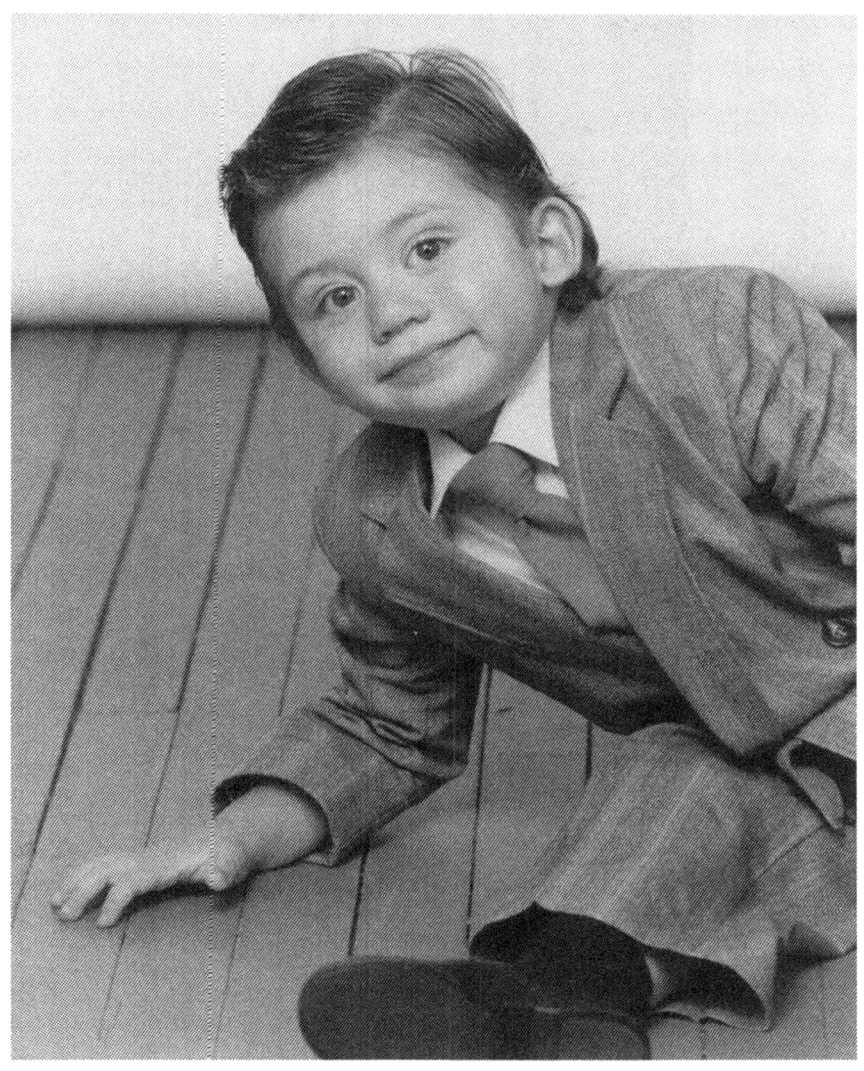

My Angel Andrei

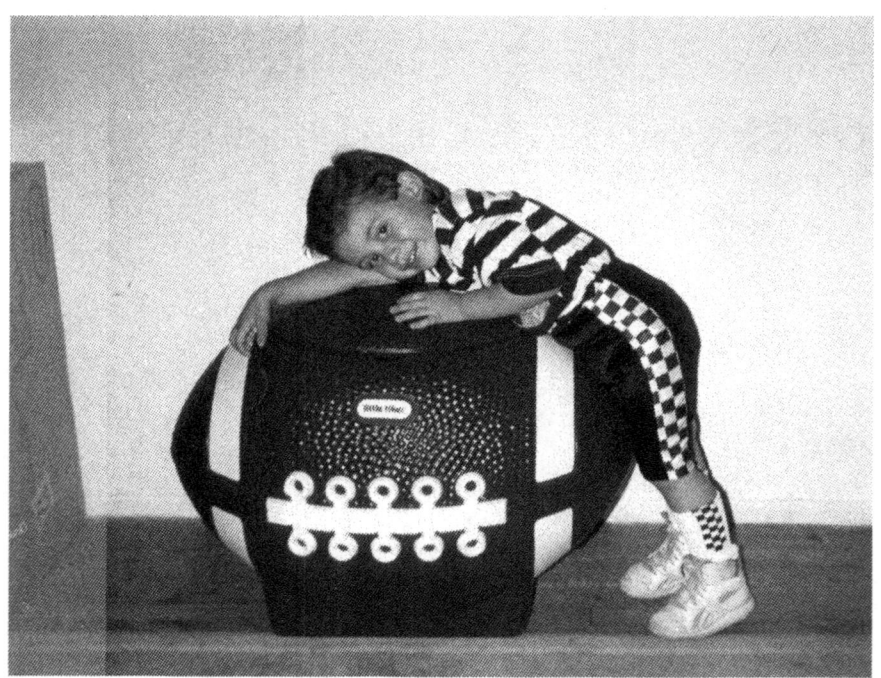

Chapter 13

Coping and Moving on

After that day, I never saw Sebastian's mother again until approximately a few months later when she was flying to Costa Rica. We approached each other and I immediately began to cry when I saw her. She embraced me and told me to please not cry, then she rapidly turned away. It appeared to be difficult for her to see me, it only brought back guilt for the pain she had caused.

I prayed everyday to find forgiveness in my heart; hatred would not allow me to be happy or find peace within myself. After a month, my boss asked me to come back to work. I later found out it was his strategy to keep me busy and preoccupied. I returned, three months after Andrei's death, Sebastian was fired. Later I applied to that department and my life began to change.

Although returning to work was helping me keep busy, it did not feel acceptable. Obviously, it made the routine, in a sense, 'normal,' but my life was far from normal. Normality and sanity would be Andrei alive, and me doing my loving duties as his mother.

I hated Sundays because it was the day he died. As Sunday approached and exactly at 7:25 p.m., that day I relived that day in my mind those unforgettable moments of Andrei's passing.

In the beginning, I began going to the cemetery almost on a daily basis, later on a weekly basis. Now I go every month or when I really feel I need to talk to him. I cried myself to sleep every night; the pain was so unbearable. I actually felt chest pains.

A very difficult time was when I first saw the headstone, it had arrived and his name was printed across it, making everything more of a reality than a bad dream. I broke down completely. Andrei's headstone has a five by seven inch photo of him imprinted on it, with a little Mickey Mouse and the Blessed Mother Mary. It also has a phrase reading; "*Andy Pandy, You Live In Our Hearts Forever, And One Day We Will Meet Again And Live Eternal Life Together.*"

Tragically, eight months after Andrei's burial, his coffin had to be exhumed because the cemetery had not buried the coffin six feet under and they were being sued. I had a Catholic priest come out to bless and pray over his coffin. It was a dreadful sight, the coffin was muddy and I knew my Andrei was in there and I could not see him. We all prayed over him and laid him back to rest. I felt I was reliving his funeral all over again. My family and close friends attended and Sebastian was informed of it through his brother, Gary. Sebastian did not appear but Gary did attend. I began to feel a numb pain in my heart trying to understand why I had to be put through this again, especially for my Andy Pandy, who should have been laid to rest.

Andrei is buried with my grandmother. On Christmas, I decorate with a miniature tree, on Easter I take him a basket with plastic colored eggs and, when I feel up to it, I take his cassette player and play for him his Disney songs. I pray over him and ask him to take care of me, to bless me and protect me from any danger. I ask Andrei to intercede with God for me, and, in some way, help me find happiness to heal my broken heart.

To assist me in my grieving process, Sister Angela had me attend a new weekly support group she established through the church. I attended and also joined an additional one called Compassionate

Friends. Both had a different style but the same subject: How to cope with losing a beloved child.

I seldom visited the therapist. I explained to her how, during the week, I would be fine but once I attended one of these support groups, I would really feel *awful*. I said I did not feel they were helping me but making me feel more depressed. I would be fine during the week and then all of sudden I was a total mess and cried uncontrollable.

She explained this was normal because, during the whole week, I kept myself so busy it prevented me from dealing with my loss. It made so much sense. During the week, I was not allowing myself to deal with it and on the days of the support group, I had to sit down and deal with the true reality of my pain. So, I sat and discussed my emotions with others empathetic to me.

This was all part of the grieving process, and it was good for me because I needed to be understood. All these other people definitely understood. I went to get a physical check up because I kept experiencing chest pains; they diagnosed it as stress-related. I thought I was having a heart attack.

I decided not to continue with the therapist because I felt she had already served her purpose. I saw her at the request of Dr. Hensley, and in order to deal with Andrei's passing. Now I was dealing with it on a daily basis; through the support groups and through much prayer, I was getting through the most painful experience of my life. I also began to read many books about life after death. These books encouraged me to believe in the beautiful life that exists after we die, and this helped me cope, knowing Andrei was in an amazing place surrounded by so much beauty and peace.

Sister Angela also involved me in teaching Sunday school to children who were about to make their first communion. I knew nothing about teaching but took the chance anyhow. It was so fulfilling, the children who were about seven, loved me. My best friend, Jennifer, and I taught the class together. We taught them their prayers and read chapters to them about the life of Christ. We also made special time for them to speak to us in private if they wanted to share any problems they felt they were having. Many children were sad because of their home situation due to parents who fought a lot. We encouraged them to pray and release their emotions to feel better. We taught the class for about a year. Then I decided to travel more and experience other cultures or, basically, run away.

*   *   *

At times, I look back at when I was so innocent and naïve about what the future might hold for me, such as love, marriage and children. I am shocked at what I have experienced as a young woman, it was not what I imagined it to be. However, I will not give up in believing I will find happiness in love, marriage and children. I can and will have it all one day, except its not complete without Andrei. He expects me to move on and does want me to be very happy, even though he is not physically with me.

I take one day at a time. There are my good days and my bad days; I am usually very upbeat and always try to be very optimistic about life. I smile and laugh a lot, and am very grateful when I can be like that because the depressing days tear me apart.

The friends I surround myself with are good people who truly care for me and listen when I need to express my emotions. They say they could never see themselves coping with what I have coped with. I tell them, "I used to believe the same and never thought I would be able to survive such a loss. My heart is missing an important piece that can never be replaced but through faith in God and prayers, the love of my family and the support of my friends. Knowing Andrei would not want me to give up, I continue in my journey and with my destiny."

I believe we think we do not have it within us to deal with such tragedy, but I also believe we do not give ourselves the credit we really deserve. We are capable of surviving; we are capable of making a negative experience positive and memorable in the best way possible. We as humans need to love, treasure and respect ourselves, look deep inside and pull out the hidden strength we carry, pray and believe God will carry us through, regardless of religious preference, we all believe in God and we all pray in similar ways. We owe it to ourselves to care and love ourselves.

We were put into this world for a purpose, make the most of it and know things happen for a reason. In the end you will become what I know I have become: strong, courageous and more knowledgeable about the purpose and lessons God wants to teach us. Although we try to bargain with God, I would pray and plead with God to allow me to keep Andrei even if he remained paralyzed; I would be content to take care of him for the rest of our lives. We must learn not to be selfish when God needs our loved ones back.

Share your love, kindness and warmth with those who want and need it. You will be pleased to know you are able to help a person in need and share what you have learned. It will help in putting closure where it is needed.

Time heals all pain, but there will be days you feel time never healed any pain. There will be a day, a holiday, an event that will trigger something inside you and it will feel as though it was just yesterday you lost your child. I see other children and something about them will help me remember something about Andrei and I begin to miss him tremendously. I listen to music, and just like persons who are suffering from a broken love affair relate to a particular song, I relate to it with my son, my broken heart.

Andrei's birthday is right after Christmas and New Years, which makes it most difficult, three holidays all at once, only a week apart. I have put up a Christmas tree once since his passing and decided I will not put one up until I have a child again and the Christmas spirit can shine brighter. It's my choice, it's what I feel to be right for me. We all have our own timing.

Two years had passed since Andrei's death and I began getting sued for unpaid hospital bills, then I had my wages held from my payroll checks. I almost had a nervous breakdown so the doctor put me on disability until my legal problems were solved; it took a bit over a year until things were resolved. I later discovered that Sebastian had gone to court and promised he would make payments on a settlement made with the collection agency, but soon after, he left the country so they came after me. However, I was very blessed by Gregory Chudacoff's generosity, an attorney and friend who assisted me in all the legal work without ever charging me for his services.

About five years after Andrei's passing, I ran into Sebastian at the airport. He was nervous and I feel he was intimidated by my maturity. After we greeted each other, I told him how my life was moving on and he told me about his. As he was getting ready to walk away, I turned to him and said, "Sebastian, I just want to tell you I forgive you for everything. I truly hope you find happiness."

It seemed as though he wanted to cry, he hugged me and kissed me on the cheek and walked away. I thought it would probably be the last time I would ever see him. For me, it was a great sense of closure; I had not seen him since the funeral and did not know how I would react after seeing him. I also needed to know what my feelings were. I knew then I did not love him anymore. The enormous love I had for him had finally vanished.

Tragically, it took Andrei's death for me to change and let go of this grand love I felt for Sebastian. If I had not experienced this loss, I honestly believe I would probably have been like a ping-pong ball back and forth in this unhealthy relationship.

He called me a few weeks after our encounter and said he was impressed with how I looked and how I continued with my life. Sebastian said he was seeing a counselor and realized he made many mistakes. One was losing me, he wished we would have married and made the most of our time with Andrei. Through counseling, he was able to express the regrets and the awareness of his controlling parents who did not allow him to live his life; he was trying to become a better person. He said how people would meet him and adore him but they just could not believe he was not attached. They were intrigued as to why he was all alone. Sebastian has a great personality and is able to make friends easily; people like him. I liked him, the nurses liked him, many liked him but, when he showed the other side of himself, it was destructive and disappointing.

About a year and half after that, he called and we began a sort of friendship, talking for many days and many hours. He said it has been very difficult for him since Andrei's passing to feel happy, he missed him a lot. I reassured him Andrei loved him very much in lieu of his absence, and he needed to be happy and not dwell on the past. I had forgiven him and I knew Andrei had also. Sebastian wanted to meet with me but he was living in San Diego and wanted to arrange for us to meet. He also wanted to come speak to my parents because he felt he owed them another apology.

I was reluctant to meet with him and made excuses; I felt I did not want to rehash the past. If my conversations on the telephone would help him find peace, I wanted to help and thus help myself understand many unanswered questions and doubts. Honestly, I would have liked to see him and talk face to face, but I realized during our many hours of conversations he had not grown as I had expected and he would bring me down. I needed to think of myself and analyze if it was going to do me good. This time around, love and youth did not blind my judgment. Finally, I saw the light at the end of the tunnel.

I asked Sebastian to stop calling me when he called me one evening and it appeared he had been drinking. As we were talking, the telephone somehow kept disconnecting as if someone was purposely doing it. I caught on when I suspected there was another person in the same room. I did not hear from Sebastian again until the next morning. I told

Sebastian I needed him to be honest with me for once, I would have more respect for him if he was able to tell me the truth.

Sebastian finally confessed there was a female friend with him who was only a "friend" and she had no idea that it was me, otherwise that incident would have not occurred. I told Sebastian in a very firm but calm voice, "Sebastian, this is not the old Antoinette that you once knew. I have changed and grown, I am a woman now! Please, she may have not known it was me, but you knew I was at the other end of the phone. And you not only allowed her to be disrespect me but you also disrespected me. I have permitted you to enter into my life once again because I wanted to help you heal and you keep hurting me. I want you never to call me again. Live your life and be happy. Goodbye! And God Bless You!"

I have heard through the grapevine that he is not happy and physically looks deteriorated. He has not married and has no other children. I honestly wish him well, I will always have a special place in my heart for Sebastian because he is Andrei's father, and we conceived him with love. But, as a man, I have no respect for him because I never saw the major changes I expected to see in him after the loss of a child. The growth and spirituality, the value of the precious life God has granted us is learned through the lessons of life we live and the value of courage, faith, survival and love we must share with each other.

Andrei, with the grace of God, came to teach us that very important lesson and his death was not in vain because my family, friends and I live and learn and are able to spread the beauty of life and forgiveness. It's all about becoming a better person and making an effort everyday to improve our imperfections and flaws.

Sebastian has not let himself grow to the fullest of his capacity and his spirituality is limited. I believe it's because he has not found it in his heart to forgive himself. When he comes to that realization, he will finally learn to live with peace within.

I saw Sebastian, his parents and sister one last time, but unfortunately under tragic circumstances. His brother Gary had passed away suddenly. I felt I needed to pay my respects and say my final goodbye to Gary. Gary was a kind, goodhearted, loving and compassionate human being. I truly loved him because Andrei and I received love, understanding and respect from him.

I was with the family during the two days the funeral was held; they treated me with respect and we all embraced and cried together. I truly empathized with their pain.

This step allowed me to focus on my feelings towards them, spending time with them during this time of their loss. I knew then I had put the past behind me and had traveled to a higher dimension of spirituality and forgiveness, followed by closure. That final day I cried a lot. I cried because I realized so vividly the fact that "We are nobody in this world, life can change so quickly and why does there have to be so much pain and hurt. We all could have made a difference if we knew how to carry our lives with humility."

Life is a mystery! The irony is that, nine years after Andrei's funeral, here we were brought back together for another funeral. It allowed us to see again how life is so vulnerable.

*   *   *

Losing Andrei was as though I had become a widow, because my life revolved around him. Taking care of him and nurturing him was part of my daily routine. I felt extremely empty and, with plenty of time on my hands, I enrolled in college and obtained my associates degree in liberal arts. When I went to receive my diploma, I held Andrei's picture in my hands; I had done this most of all for him. Words can't express how I felt – he was my only child. Children are supposed to outlive their parents, not the other way around. I believe my son's life was prolonged because of the grace of God, state-of-the-art technology, and because he felt the need to hold on until I was strong enough to accept his departure from this world.

I look back at the unforgettable times we shared his courage, strength, his manliness, and his desire to survive. I reflect upon all this and it keeps me going from one day to the next. Knowing he would not want me to give up, I am a survivor. As strong as I have become, I am also aware that everyday I grow more and try to become a better person on a daily basis. I realized I needed to make more drastic changes; Andrei's room had remained the same with the only exception of adding a treadmill to it. My thought was I would leave the room the same until I left my home to marry and begin a new transition in my life. Then I would put the belongings away to begin a new life.

It took eight years (1998) for me after Andrei's passing to actually let go and allow him to rest in peace. My love for my child is so grand that, although I had believed I had accepted his departure, my subconscious felt I was betraying him if I put away his belongings and he was being forgotten. I love my Andrei so much that I wanted to feel his presence with his belongings surrounding me.

I decided to return to therapy and try to find a way to let go but not feel I was betraying his memory. Within three months, I successfully accomplished just that. We practiced imagery and envisioned myself with Andrei during his birth, growing years and illness. We later discussed his death and how I did everything possible to give him the proper care. I cried as many tears as though I had just buried him. A lot of healing remained to be done and apparently, I had not completely let go. The imagery also consisted of putting away his belongings and going through that pain before actually doing it.

I was aware that, during Andrei's illness, I did not allow myself to cry because I wanted to be strong. Since his memory was so vivid to me, I needed to finally fully mourn his death. I felt a lot of sadness, and my emotions felt the pain of losing a child and coming to terms with never seeing him again. I would not have the blessing of watching him grow and follow his dreams.

I chose Andrei's birthday, January 4th, to be the day of a new birth of my new life and release of the past. Never forgetting, but forgiving him for leaving me behind!

With the help, love and support of my beautiful mother who has always been there for me, we began to transform the room's appearance. I played the Frank Sinatra greatest hits CD in memory of Andrei, and we began packing his stuffed animals and toys. All was going well until I got to the clothes. Andrei enjoyed carrying coins in his pockets and, as I packed his clothes, I gathered a red sweatshirt full of coins in the right-hand pocket. I burst into tears, he had touched those coins and kept them in his pocket. My Andy was gone forever.

Every weekend, my mother and sister helped me finish putting away the belongings, storing the ones I wanted to keep in the garage and pack the ones I was going to donate. After painting the room, I remodeled the furnishings and now I have the satisfaction of an adult room with the proper décor to make me comfortable. I know Andrei is still with me, I feel his presence in the room and his smell. I continue to feel sad at times, in particular the anniversary date of his passing. However, it's a different kind of sadness, I feel acceptance and peace but I do miss him.

*   *   *

Several incidents occurred before I finally returned to therapy and stopped feeling sorry for myself. I interpret these as signs for my future.

One day I was extremely depressed. I felt lonely and very sad, and I picked up a picture of his that was on the table in Andrei's room. It showed him with all the tubes connected to his body, the oxygen tank beside him and yet wearing a big smile. I said to myself, *Well, in lieu of his condition he always looked at life 'happy'*. I knew Andrei looked at life as I taught him to look at it: optimistically.

I said to myself and to Andrei, " I will hang in there, I won't give up on you or myself."

I started to walk away when suddenly his Mickey Mouse music toy, which had been turned off for months, rang loudly. I got chills down my spine and went crying to my mother in the kitchen to tell her what had just happened. While telling her, my father went quickly to the room and said out loud, "Andrei, why do you give your mother signs and not me."

As my dad was walking away the toy rang, and my dad cried. Andrei has not abandoned us, he is spiritually with us and he will not abandon us. I had told him the day of his Rosary at his coffin to always give me a sign he was around so that life could be easier to bear. He has been granting my request.

Another beautiful incident was when I went with my friends to Costa Rica for a vacation. We went river rafting and were supposed to put us in a beginners' level expedition but, for whatever mistake or misunderstanding, we were put in the advance level group. Obviously, we did not find out until we were in the river. My friends and I were so scared; at one point, I began to pray and pleaded with Andrei to give me a sign that he was with us. I asked that he throw a leaf from the tree that was pretty far away.

Five minutes later, my friend, Mariana, looked at me, pointed to my feet and said, "Look! There is a leaf on your shoe."

Tears came down into my eyes and Mariana was confused until I had the chance to tell her later about my request to Andrei.

Andrei is always spiritually with me and, through signs, he lets me become aware of his presence.

My father had open-heart surgery in 1995, due to his age and diabetes he was in critical condition. The forty eight hours following would be the most crucial if he was going to pull through. We prayed and, ironically, we were at the same hospital where Andrei passed away. It also was during the anniversary of his passing. When my father woke from the anesthesia, he said through tears that he had seen Andrei and a little friend with him walking around the bed, watching over his Tata. He was there to take care of him and Dad successfully made it through.

I had another experience that I feel is a reminder of the vulnerability of life. During a physical exam, three tumors were detected in my breasts. I underwent a mammogram and ultrasound. It appeared the tumors looked solid, and surgery to remove them as well as a biopsy would be able to detect if it was cancer. I was numb and I just kept remembering how my life changed overnight with Andrei. I was given a handbook about chemotherapy, wigs, radiation, oncologists and mastectomy. When I walked out of the hospital I began to cry uncontrollably, I walked in the street dazed, unaware of those around me. I was imagining the worst and most of all I was going to relive the pain of cancer. If I get a painful headache, I think of Andrei's pain with the tumor, and my headache does not even compare to the actuality of his pain.

As I was walking, distraught, I saw a church at the corner. I went inside and kneeled down to cry, there were people around but it did not matter to me. I said to God, "God, if this is what you want for me to experience, I accept this, but please bring back the old Antoinette who is strong and courageous, not this scared little girl. I will accept what you bring to me but just help me be strong."

I honestly prayed from the bottom of my heart and soul and, by the next day, I had come to terms with losing my hair and the possibility of losing my breasts. I told my mother who was so scared that I wanted to make a will and was prepared for the worst. I did not want to be negative, just realistic, if things did not turn out as we hoped for or what was meant to be. I was at peace with God and myself. I allowed myself to put my entire life in His hands so that "His will, thy will be done."

The following days I underwent bilateral breast lumpectomies and waited for the results. Thanks be to God, the tumors were not cancerous and, in actuality, were similar to cysts.

Once again, the experience allowed me to grow spiritually and finally let go of any doubts about life. At last, I have made my peace with God; I know He loves me and everything we experience and encounter throughout our lives has a significant, valid purpose.

I realized again not to question everything, but live the experience and grow from it. Each time we become wiser and spiritually connected with God and ourselves. It allows us to savor life to the fullest and we are able to share with others the significance of living each day at a time. Life gives us signs as reminders to value life and we need to detect them, slow down and make the necessary changes in our busy schedules.

Chapter 14

Cancer Research

Nine years after Andrei's death, the research department at the University of Southern California sent me a consent form to be signed so that Andrei's tumor could be studied for tests. The USC Research Department had been hired by the American Cancer Society to study the tumor of Chordoma. They indicate that, in ten years, only seventy-four cases have been reported. Only four of those were in children, Andrei being one of them. Ultimately, the study would prove if it has an environmental or genetic influence.

Multiple questions about family health history had to be answered in order to assist the studies. I was able to obtain Sebastian's sister's address and had the research department mail the sheets under her care, but addressed to Sebastian. The department will keep me informed on all research and studies in much detail. I pray this will help other children, to find an answer to this horrific tumor and other lives may be saved.

I am happy to know this research study is taking place because there was no protocol to treat this type of rare tumor. The information about this rare tumor was limited and this will definitely expand their knowledge. Maybe I will also get the opportunity to become acquainted with other parents whose child has been a victim of this disease.

I also sent the research team an eight by ten inch photo of Andrei, so that they can put a face with the name. The coordinator sent me a pleasant letter in response, and left a telephone message on my recorder, letting me know she was very touched and it made an enormous difference.

Chapter 15
My Message to You

As I've said, life should be appreciated and treasured immensely, enjoyed everyday to its fullest for there may be no tomorrow. Everything we do in life revolves around the morals, values and the humane quality within us. Decisions and the way we decide to live our lives reflect our particular nature of a human being. I believe it all starts with us as children, obviously our parents' role is the most significant. They instill beliefs, goodness and kindness to be part of ourselves, which we should practice and be able to integrate with others whom we encounter in our daily lives.

I am a different person because of this experience. I would go through it all over again to have had the privilege to be Andrei's mother and be loved as I was by my son. I hope and pray that one day I will meet a good man who will value me, and one day have other children. I know Andrei is watching over me and I feel his presence many times; he has left me physically, but spiritually, he is with me.

My humble advice to those parents who are having this painful experience, is to be very strong and courageous. Do not give up or your child will sense it and he or she will give up. Be a positive influence in their lives and trust in the Lord that He will help you get through this. There will be those days of much distress and days when you will feel envious of other parents fortunate and blessed to have their children become healed or cured. You won't like what you feel inside but, through prayer and time, you will be comforted and you will be happy that at least one more child made it, even if it was not yours. These feeling are natural and it takes time to understand these emotions. As parents, it's natural that we become selfish and want to keep our child with us.

Never give up on your true feelings and your intuition. If your gut tells you something does not feel or sound right, follow it. Doctors do not know it all, it's your child and he cannot fend for himself so you need to do it. It's your obligation and responsibility as a parent to pursue medical tests although they say there is nothing medically wrong. Persist and continue obtaining second opinions until you get the right answers. If you do not persist, it might be too late for your child and he or she may not get the chance he or she deserves.

We carried our child within us for nine months. We have a bond unlike anything else, and we know our children well. I kept being told it was a psychological problem. I thank God for the courage I had to follow my heart.

I also thank God for giving me the courage to accept the things I can't change and wisdom to know the difference. I thank Him for my life and the new opportunity I now have to be happy and find peace within myself.

I go on now day by day and make it an effort to enjoy that day to the fullest. When I catch myself going too fast I try to slow it down and remember life must be treasured. I try not to procrastinate and have begun doing the things I have always wanted to do. I purchased a guitar and started taking lessons. I take kick-boxing classes as well as travel to the countries I have always wanted to visit. I feel that I am grounded, know what I want out of life, and am pursuing my goals. When I have a family of my own and a caring and loving husband, I will finally feel complete.

Chapter 16
Inspirational Poems

Although God lent our child to us, He will take our children when He feels it's time and their purpose in this world is finished. A nurse gave me the following poem:

For All Parents....

"I'll lend you for a little time, a child of mine,"
He said,
"For you to love while he lives, and mourn when
he is dead.
"It may be six or seven years, or twenty-two or three,
"But will you, till I call him back, take care of
him for me?
"He'll bring his charms to gladden you, and shall
his stay be brief,
"You'll have his lovely memories as solace for
your grief.
"I cannot promise he will stay, since all from earth
return,
"But there are lessons taught down there I want
this child to learn.

"I've looked the wide world over in my search for
teachers true,
"And from the throngs that crowd life's lane, I
have selected you.
"Now will you give him all your love, nor think
the labor vain,
"Nor hate me when I come to call, to take him
back again.
"I fancied that I heard them say, Dear Lord, Thy
will be done.
"For all the joy thy child shall bring, the risk of
grief we'll run.
"We'll shelter him with tenderness, we'll love him
while we may;
"And for the happiness we've known, will ever
grateful stay.
"But shall the angels call for him much sooner
than we planned,
"We'll brave the bitter grief that comes, and try
to understand!"

—Anonymous. West Palm Beach

If it is God's will, your child will heal but it is His will to take him.
Make certain they are the most beautiful and treasured memories of
love, that you will have no regrets of making the best of times, shared in
special love and bonding with each other. Our family, our friends, and
the special nurses who care for our children will help us deal with these
difficult times. After the turmoil, whatever results we have, depending
on our fate and destiny, we can still be winners.

We walk away as an amazing *survivor* and, after going through this,
everything else seems so insignificant. We will treasure life in a very spe-

cial way; our child touched and changed us in a way no other person would have.

They watch over us, protecting us from harm in the presence of God. We know they are at peace and although they miss us tremendously, they stay with us in a spiritual way, close to their mommies and daddies and loved ones. They had beautiful unconditional love from their parents and we had their love and tenderness. It was special to have loved them once than never to have loved or given birth to them.

Although shedding many tears from our enormous loss, it was worth every moment in our lives to experience this type of cherished love. God Bless!

The Butterfly

A man found a cocoon of a butterfly. One day
a small opening appeared, and he sat and
watched the butterfly as it struggled for several
hours to force its body through the little hole.
Then it seemed to stop making any progress.
It appeared that it had gotten as far as it could.

The man decided to help the butterfly, so he
took a pair of scissors and snipped off the
remaining bit of cocoon. The butterfly then
emerged easily, but it had a swollen body and
small, shriveled wings.

The man continued to watch the butterfly
because he expected that, at any moment, the
wings would expand and be able to support
the body, which would contract in time.

Neither happened! In fact, the butterfly spent
it's whole life crawling around with a swollen
body and shriveled wings. It was never able to fly.
What the man, in kindness and haste, did not
understand was that the restricting cocoon and
the struggle required to get through the tiny
opening were God's way of forcing fluid from
the body of the butterfly into its wings so that
it would be ready for flight once it achieved
freedom.

Sometimes struggles are exactly what we need in our life. If God allowed us to go through life without obstacles, it would cripple us. We would not be as strong as we could have been,

And.....................we would never fly.

Light

his name is Andrei, our hearts' desire
heaven's his temple, God's empire
he is Andrei, and truth is his crown
the essence of light, silence profound
wisdom is light, understanding a guide s his crown
strength a pedestal, he shines it with pride
come to it and he'll give to you
a love so sweet, a love so true
light is warm, as he is so
his name is Andrei and he'd like you to know
he is gentle, wise and meek
serene and peaceful, slow to speak
he is spirit, the idea of love
he is peace, his symbol's a dove
grace is his glory, radiant from within
he is an angel, his mother's best friend
Andrei is innocence, aged in his youth
he is the way, the light and the truth.

Navid Daniel Rastein, M.D.

Remember Me

To the living,
I am gone.
To the sorrowful,
I will never return.
To the angry,
I was cheated.
But to the happy,
I am at peace.
And to the faithful,
I have never left.
I cannot speak,
But I can listen
I cannot be seen,
But I can be heard.
So as you stand upon a shore,
Gazing at a beautiful sea—
Remember me.
As you look upon a flower,
And admire its simplicity—
Remember me.
Remember me in your heart,
Your thoughts,
And your memories,
Of the times we loved,
The times we cried,
The times we fought,

My Angel Andrei

The times we laughed.
For if you always think of me,
I will have never gone.

Anonymous.

Antoinette Romero

Safely Home

I am home in Heaven, dear ones:
Oh, so happy and so bright!
There is perfect joy and beauty
In this everlasting light.

All the pain and grief is over,
Every restless tossing passed;
I am now at peace forever,
Safely home in Heaven at last.

Did you wonder I so calmly
Trod the valley of the shade?
Oh! But Jesus' love illumined
Every dark and fearful glade.

And He came Himself to meet me
In that way so hard to tread;
And with Jesus' arm to lean on,
Could I have one doubt or dread?

Then you must not grieve so sorely,
For I love you dearly still:
Try to look beyond earth's shadows,
Pray to trust our Father's Will.

There is work still waiting for you,
So you must not idly stand;
Do it now, while life remaineth—
You shall rest in Jesus' land.

My Angel Andrei

When that work is all completed,
He will gently call you Home;
Oh, the rapture of that meeting,
Oh, the joy to see you come!

When I Must Leave You

When I must leave you for a little while

Please do not grieve and shed wild tears

And hug your sorrow to you
    Through the years.

But start out bravely with a
    Gallant smile;

And for my sake and in my name

Live on and do all things the same,

Feed not your loneliness on empty days,

But fill each waking hour in useful ways,

Reach out your hand in comfort
    And in cheer

And in turn will comfort you

And hold you near;

And never, never be afraid to die,

For I am waiting for you in the sky!

Listen With Your Heart

Memories are a treasure
time cannot take away…
So may you be surrounded
by happy ones today…
May all the love and tenderness
of golden years well spent
Come back today to fill your heart
with beauty and content…
And may you walk down MEMORY LANE
And meet the one you love
For awhile you cannot see him,
he'll be watching from above…
And if you trust your dreaming
your faith will make it true…
And if you listen with your heart
he'll come and talk with you…
So for his sake be happy
and show him that his love
Has proven strong and big enough
to reach down from above…
And you will never walk alone
when Memory's Door swings wide…
For you'll find that your beloved
is always at your side.

Comes The Dawn

After awhile you learn the subtle difference
Between holding a hand and chaining a soul,
And you learn that love doesn't mean leaning
And company doesn't mean security,
And you begin to learn that kisses aren't contracts
And presents aren't promises,
And you begin to accept your defeats
With your head up and your eyes open,
And learn to build all your roads
On today because tomorrow's ground
Is too uncertain for plans, and futures have
A way of falling down mid-flight,
After awhile you learn that even sunshine
Burns if you get too much.
So you plant your own garden and decorate
Your own soul, instead of waiting
For someone to bring you flowers,
And you learn that you really can endure…
That you really are strong
And you really do have worth.
And you learn and learn…
With every goodbye you learn.

(this poem was given to us by a patient-
we don't know the author.)

I Asked God

I asked God to take away my pride,
    and God said, "No."
He said it was not form him to take away
    but for me to give up.
I asked God to make my handicapped child whole,
    and God said, "No."
He said his spirit is whole,
    his body is only temporary.
I asked God to grant me patience,
    and God said, 'No."
He said that patience is a by-product of tribulation;
    It isn't granted, it earned.
I asked God to give me happiness,
and God said, "No."
He said He gives blessings;
    happiness is up to me.
I asked God to make my spirit grow
and God said "No."
He said I must grow on my own,
    but He will prune me to make me fruitful.
I asked God if he loves me,
    and God said, "Yes."
He gave His only Son who died for me,
    and I will be in heaven some day because I believe.
I asked God to help me love others,
    and God said, "Ah, finally you have the idea."

Antoinette Romero

To Those I Have Loved

To those I have loved and to those who loved me,
        when I am gone release me; let me go.
I have so many things to see and do,
        you must not tie yourself to me with tears.
Be happy that we had so many years.

I gave you my love you can only guess,
        how much you gave me happiness.
I thank you for the love you each have shown,
        but now it's time I travel on alone.

So grieve awhile for me if grieve you must.
        Then let your grief be comforted by trust.
It's only for awhile that we must part,
        so bless the memories within your heart.

I won't be far away for life goes on,
        so if you need me call and I will come.
Though you can't see or touch me I'll be near,
        and if you listen within your heart you'll hear
        all my love around you soft and clear.

And then when you must come this way alone,
I'll greet you with a smile and welcome you home.

Author's Biography

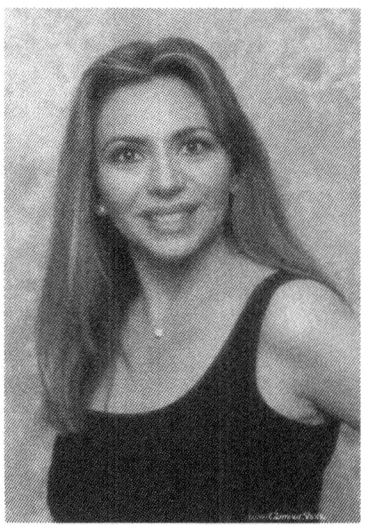

Antoinette Romero was born in Long Beach, California. Parents are natives of Guaymas, Sonora, Mexico. Antoinette, currently resides in Southern California and will soon pursue a degree in psychology.

E-mail *MyAngelAndrei@yahoo.com* to share your thoughts and feelings with the author.

www.ingramcontent.com/pod-product-compliance
Lightning Source LLC
Chambersburg PA
CBHW061310280526
45784CB00002B/953